THE SCID-D INTERVIEW
DISSOCIATION ASSESSMENT
IN THERAPY, FORENSICS, AND RESEARCH

MARLENE STEINBERG, M.D.

Client's Identifier: _____   ID No.: _____

Interviewer: _____   Interviewer ID: _____

Study: _____   Study No.: _____

Evaluation: ○ Initial   Rater is: ○ Interviewer

○ Reevaluation   ○ Observer

Date of Interview: _____
(Mo./Day/Year)

Consultation with: _____   Time Interview Began: _____

Ended: _____

With this new edition, the acronym "SCID-D" stands for Semi-Structured Clinical Interview for Dissociative Symptoms and Disorders.

The correct citation for this book is: Steinberg M: *The SCID-D: Dissociation Assessment in Therapy, Forensics, and Research.* Washington, DC, American Psychiatric Association Publishing, 2023

Manufactured in the United States of America on acid-free paper

26 25 24 23 22   5 4 3 2 1

American Psychiatric Association Publishing
800 Maine Avenue, S.W.
Suite 900
Washington, D.C. 20024
www.appi.org

ISBN 978-1-61537-342-0

CONTENTS

Acknowledgments...v

Key Points About the SCID-D...vii

Preface to the 2023 Edition..ix

PART I: PSYCHIATRIC AND MEDICAL HISTORY 1

History Questions 3

PART II: THE FIVE COMPONENTS OF DISSOCIATION ASSESSMENT 17

Amnesia: Past and Current Symptoms..19

Amnesia refers to a subjective sense of gaps in one's memory for autobiographical information or experiences, or for blocks of time that have passed, where such lapses cannot be attributed to ordinary forgetfulness.

Depersonalization: Past and Current Symptoms...29

Depersonalization refers to a feeling of disconnection from one's self (e.g., from one's feelings, thoughts, behavior, or body), or a sense of being an outside observer of one's self.

Derealization: Past and Current Symptoms...39

Derealization refers to a feeling of disconnection from one's surroundings (e.g., people or surroundings feel as if they are unfamiliar, unreal, or distorted).

Identity Confusion: Past and Current Symptoms...45

Identity confusion refers to subjective feelings of uncertainty, puzzlement, conflict, or struggle regarding one's own identity or sense of self.

Identity Alteration: Past and Current Symptoms...49

Identity alteration refers to observable behavior associated with alterations or shifts in one's identity or personality states.

PART III: FURTHER EXPLORATION OF IDENTITY CONFUSION & ALTERATION 57

Associated Features of Identity Confusion and Identity Alteration..........................59

Mood Changes; Flashbacks; Internal Dialogues, Voices, and Intrusive Thoughts 59

Follow-Up Sections: Identity Confusion and Alteration 65

Parts of Self and Identity Confusion Follow-Up 67

Mood Changes Follow-Up 73

Depersonalization Follow-Up..77

Different Names Follow-Up 81

Voices, Dialogues, and Intrusive Thoughts Follow-Up 87

Childlike Part Follow-Up 91

Flashback Follow-Up...95

Different Person Follow-Up 101

Possession or Trance Follow-Up 105

ICD-11-Specific Follow-Up: DID versus Partial DID 111

DSM-5-TR Specific: Optional History Questions Relevant to Other Specified Dissociative Disorder (OSDD), Example 2 115

Citation: Steinberg M: The SCID-D: Dissociation Assessment in Therapy, Forensics, and Research. Washington, DC, American Psychiatric Association Publishing, 2023

PART IV: Post-Interview Ratings 117

   Nonverbal/Observable Cues... 119

     Behaviors and symptoms observed during the interview that, if present, can provide additional evidence in support of a dissociative disorder diagnosis.

APPENDICES

Appendix 1: SCID-D Severity Rating Definitions 123

Appendix 2: Typical SCID-D Symptom Profiles for the Dissociative Disorders 135

Appendix 3A: ICD-11 Diagnostic Criteria for the Dissociative Disorders............. 139

Appendix 3B: DSM-5-TR Diagnostic Criteria for the Dissociative Disorders...... 151

Appendix 4A: Summary Scoresheet (with ICD-11 diagnoses) 159

Appendix 4B: Summary Scoresheet (with DSM-5-TR diagnoses) 163

Appendix 4C: Charting The Client's SCID-D Profile 167

ACKNOWLEDGMENTS

For their ongoing support, shared expertise, and recommendations related to the 2023 edition of the SCID-D, I am grateful for the advice of expert colleagues Drs. Daniel Brown, Diane Sholomskas, Pamela Hall, Olivier Piedfort-Marin, and Mr. Remy Aquarone. I'd also like to express my gratitude to Olivier Piedfort-Marin and Mr. Remy Aquarone for their recommendations about making the SCID-D more applicable for our international colleagues using ICD-11.

Having received both a First Independent Research Support and Transition Award and a Research Project Grant (R01) from the National Institute of Mental Health (NIMH), I conducted field trials and other SCID-D research at Yale University School of Medicine over a span of nine years. The field trials would not have been possible without the support of my mentors and research collaborators, including Jack Maser, Ph.D., at the NIMH and the late Drs. Bruce Rounsaville, Domenic Cicchetti, and Robert Spitzer, who served as a consultant to this grant. I am grateful for the shared expertise and nurturing support from the late Reverend Ollie Hall and Dr. Daniel Brown. Thanks is also due to Josephine Buchanan, SCID-D Research Coordinator, and my staff, Jonathan Lovins, Sue Macary, Gerald Melnick, and Karen Zych, as well as a team of empathically attuned interviewers: Christine Amis, Jean Bancroft, Susan Davis, Pamela Hall, Marie Matheson, Geanine Peck, and Susan Wharfe. In addition, I'd like to thank all my colleagues who have generously shared their expertise, who participated in SCID-D multicenter field trials or who furthered SCID-D education: Drs. Elizabeth Bowman, Philip Coons, Catherine Fine, David Fink, Francine Howland, Richard Kluft, George Mahl, and Charles Rousell.

My research stands on the shoulders of clinical researchers whose pioneering phenomenological work in the field of dissociation influenced and paved the way for the SCID-D, including, but not limited to, Elizabeth Bowman, Philip Coons, George Fraser, Richard Kluft, Frank Putnam, and the late Jack and Helen Watkins. There are also many clinicians and researchers worldwide I wish to thank, who, through their use of the SCID-D in research and clinical practice, have contributed to SCID-D clinical applications and psychometrics and further advanced our understanding, diagnosis, and treatment of dissociation cross-culturally. These include Drs. Bethany Brand, J.M. Darves-Bornoz, Nel Draijer, George Fraser, Ursula Gast, Heather Gingrich, Ellen Kjaerulff Jepsen, Helge Knudsen, Christoph Mueller-Pfeiffer, Ellert Nijenhuis, F. Rodewald, Vedat Sar, Eli Somer, and Ken Welburn. I'd also like to thank the members of the New England Study Group for Dissociation, including Drs. Anthony Fons, Bruce Levi, Carol Pulice, and Ruth and Bart Schofield.

I am grateful to my publisher, John McDuffie, for ongoing support of my work, and to Greg Kuny and the entire production staff at American Psychiatric Association Publishing. Nicolas Taylor, Terri Morgan, and Stephen Grigelevich have all been a pleasure to work with in creating and compiling this new edition. I continue to be inspired by my husband and research collaborator, Peter Ward, whose expertise in law, dissociation, and statistical analysis has been invaluable and enriched SCID-D research. Finally, I wish to thank participants in the SCID-D field trials, who graciously shared their lived experiences of dissociation with the hope that others would not suffer years of misdiagnosis as they had.

KEY POINTS ABOUT THE SCID-D

1. Dissociation is the mind's way of coping with overwhelming stress and trauma, characterized by a sense of disconnection from one's self, other people, or one's surroundings. Given the ubiquity of trauma, the assessment of dissociation is essential for accurate diagnosis and trauma-informed treatment.

2. The SCID-D is an interactive, semistructured interview for assessing dissociation in adults and adolescents based on Dr. Steinberg's innovative Five Component Model of Dissociation Assessment. By guiding clinicians, step-by-step, in systematically exploring and assessing the Model's five primary components, the SCID-D yields rich, clinically relevant information about a person's inner world and lived experience. This provides a framework for understanding an individual's sense of disconnection from their authentic feelings and needs.

3. The Model's five primary components are amnesia, depersonalization, derealization, identity confusion, and identity alteration. Each component is multifaceted in presentation, occurring along a spectrum of severity, and each represents an adaptive survival mechanism employed in the face of adverse life experiences. Particular dissociative disorders correspond to distinct mixtures of severity levels for each of the five components ranging from normative to problematic, as specified by applying the SCID-D's severity rating definitions.

4. Dissociative symptoms and disorders are commonly underdiagnosed, in part because they often occur outside of an individual's conscious awareness. When dissociative symptoms are misattributed as due solely to depression, anxiety, psychosis, addictions, attention problems, or posttraumatic stress disorder, failure to diagnose the underlying dissociative disorder can lead to higher rates of hospitalization and suicide attempts, and prolonged suffering. Early and accurate detection of dissociation using the SCID-D reduces these risks.

5. Although presentations of overt manifestations of dissociative symptoms may vary by culture, the Five Component Model of Dissociation Assessment as applied by the SCID-D interview yields diagnostic results that have proven to be culturally invariant, providing a universally applicable means for detecting underlying dissociative conditions.

6. Over thirty years of worldwide research and clinical use have confirmed the good to excellent interrater reliability and validity of the SCID-D interview and its implementation of the Five Component Model of Dissociation Assessment. The interview has demonstrated a powerful ability to distinguish people with dissociative symptoms and disorders from those with other conditions, and is widely regarded as the gold standard in the field. This 2023 edition of the SCID-D includes all the psychometrically validated interview questions of previous editions, preserving its good-to-excellent psychometric properties.

Cite as: Steinberg M: The SCID-D Interview: Dissociation Assessment in Therapy, Forensics, and Research.
Washington, DC, American Psychiatric Association Publishing, 2023

7. Somatic symptoms (e.g., pseudoseizures, functional movement symptoms) are common manifestations of underlying dissociative disorders. When patients with such symptoms are assessed with the SCID-D, often a more complex dissociative disorder will be detected, superseding the somatic symptom diagnosis initially suggested by ICD or DSM. Establishing the patient's true dissociative condition facilitates treatment aimed at recovery, not just somatic symptom amelioration.

8. The SCID-D's method of evaluation is independent of DSM or ICD nosology, though its results can be mapped into their diagnostic criteria.

9. In addition to its diagnostic utility, the interview has been found to provide therapeutic benefits, both in accelerating the therapeutic relationship and eliciting material about a patient's inner world, especially when administered by a nonjudgmental, empathic interviewer. Moreover, the interview's results can provide a roadmap for patient healing, especially through interviewer feedback.

10. The SCID-D is compatible with nearly all therapeutic approaches. Designed to elicit information about an individual's sense of self, the SCID-D's results are particularly well suited to therapeutic models predicated upon multiple aspects of self, including Compassion-Focused Therapy, Ego State Therapy, Internal Family Systems, Schema Therapy, and Phase Oriented Trauma and Dissociation Informed Treatment.

Administering and scoring the SCID-D interview requires familiarity with the procedures outlined in the *Interviewer's Guide to the SCID-D*, either the 1993 edition or the expanded 2023 edition under development.

PREFACE TO THE 2023 EDITION

Dissociation is the mind's way of coping with overwhelming stress and trauma. Facing what it perceives as a life-threatening situation, the mind disconnects from its immediate surroundings, compartmentalizing authentic feelings—like despair or terror—that may hinder survival. At some point in their lives, to some degree, most people have experienced dissociation. For instance, following a car accident or the death of a loved one, you might feel emotionally numb or disconnected. This transient dissociation usually isn't problematic. But when due to trauma that's severe or ongoing, dissociation can cause considerable distress and/or difficulty functioning. Children, adolescents, and adults exposed to attachment traumas, neglect, or abuse, as well as combat veterans and survivors of sexual assault, are all at risk for developing recurrent dissociation—with the attendant and abiding feelings of inner fragmentation, self-alienation, shame, and fear. It is important to note that trauma encompasses more than might come to mind at first. For example, in addition to physical or sexual abuse, underrecognized traumas, such as chronic childhood invalidation, vicarious trauma, or intergenerational trauma, can also contribute to the development of dissociation.

Over the last few decades, societal consciousness has come to recognize the high prevalence of trauma in the public.[1] A study by the National Survey of Children's Health found that almost 50% of children under the age of 17 in the United States have experienced at least one significant trauma (The Child and Adolescent Health Measurement Initiative 2017–2018). What's more, a growing number of clinicians have endorsed therapy models predicated upon multiple aspects of self,[2] suggesting the wide prevalence of inner fragmentation typical of persons who have suffered trauma. Still, very few survivors ever learn that what they're suffering from is called *dissociation*, despite the fact that it underlies all posttraumatic conditions. Simply put, "all trauma-related disorders (i.e., Acute Stress Disorder, PTSD, and Dissociative Disorders) share a common central psychobiological pathology that is dissociative" (Van der Hart, Nijenhuis, and Steele 2005).

---

[1] Dr. Vedat Sar reviewed an extensive body of epidemiological research to investigate the prevalence of dissociative disorders. Typically correlated with childhood abuse and other traumas, dissociative disorders, Sar concludes, "constitute a hidden and neglected public health problem," with around 10% of clinical populations, and 0.4%–3% of the general population, suffering from Dissociative Identity Disorder (DID) (Sar 2011). (Prevalence is even higher when all dissociative conditions, not just DID, are considered. For more information, see Johnson, Cohen, Kasen, and Brook 2006, a major epidemiological study of dissociative disorders in the community.)

[2] Such models include Compassion-Focused Therapy, Ego State Therapy, Internal Family Systems Therapy, Phase Oriented Trauma and Dissociation Informed Treatment, Structural Dissociation, and other integrative models (Brown and Eliot 2016; Fine 1996; Fisher 2017; Gilbert 2010; Herman 2015; Howell 2020; International Society for the Study of Trauma and Dissociation 2005; Kluft 1993; Kluft, Bloom, and Kinzie 2000; Perry and Dobson 2013; Schwartz 2001; Siegel 2020; Sinason 2010; Steele, Van der Hart, and Nijenhuis 2005; Van der Hart, Nijenhuis, and Steele 2006; Watkins and Watkins 1997).

Cite as: Steinberg M: The SCID-D Interview: Dissociation Assessment in Therapy, Forensics, and Research. Washington, DC, American Psychiatric Association Publishing, 2023

The connection between posttraumatic stress disorder (PTSD) and dissociation deserves emphasis, with empirical research illuminating a robust correlation.[3] In recognition of the prevalence of a limited subset of dissociative symptoms (specifically depersonalization and derealization) in people suffering from PTSD, DSM-5 added a dissociative subtype of PTSD, marking a watershed moment in the PTSD field's understanding of these afflictions (American Psychiatric Association 2013). Recent studies have noted a significant percentage of persons with PTSD with histories of childhood and/or adult trauma met criteria for the dissociative subtype, ranging from 54% to 83% (Hill, Wolff, Bigony et al. 2019; Swart, Wildschut, Draijer et al. 2020).

There is a growing body of empirical evidence indicating that many PTSD sufferers experience a range of dissociative symptoms beyond depersonalization or derealization, and that the new dissociative subtype of PTSD may understate dissociation's role in PTSD. Studies that evaluated the full range of dissociative symptoms found that 34%–87% of people suffering from PTSD met the criteria for a dissociative disorder, many with dissociative conditions beyond what is detectable using diagnostic tools for the dissociative subtype of PTSD (Darves-Bornoz 1997; Darves-Bornoz, Degiovanni, and Gaillard 1995; Darves-Bornoz, Berger, Degiovanni et al. 1999; Roca, Hart, Kimbrell 2006). Vietnam veterans diagnosed with PTSD were found not only to suffer from the full range and severity of dissociative symptoms but also to have dissociative symptom severity scores that were virtually identical to those of persons suffering from complex dissociative disorders (Bremner, Steinberg, Southwick et al. 1993). In light of this research, some experts have asserted that "dissociation is characteristic of all PTSD" (Dorahy and Van der Hart 2015). Elizabeth Howell speaks for a growing number of experts in boldly defining trauma as "that which causes dissociation" (Howell 2020).

When someone suffers from dissociation, it is not usually their presenting complaint. Extensive research indicates that people suffering from dissociation seek treatment for depression, anxiety, mood swings, hearing voices, attention problems, obsessive-compulsive symptoms, addictions, self-destructive behavior, and somatic symptoms—essentially everything *but* dissociation (Bailey, Boyer, Brand 2019; Bakim, Baran, Diyaddin et al. 2016; Bowman 2006; Coons 1984; Coons, Bowman, Milstein 1988; Goff, Jenike, Baer et al. 1992; Haugen and Castillo 1999; Karadag, Sar, Tamar-Gurol et al. 2005; Kluft 1985, 1987; Nijenhuis 2000; Putnam, Guroff, Silberman et al. 1986; Sar 2011; Sar, Kundakci, Kiziltan et al. 2003; Somer, Altusa, and Ginzburg 2010; Steinberg 1995; Steinberg and Schnall 2010; Steinberg, Barry, Sholomskas et al. 2005; Tanner, Wyss, Perron et al. 2017). Yet optimal care depends on accurate diagnosis. For decades, lack of a reliable methodology for diagnosing dissociation led to misdiagnosis, ineffective treatment, and unnecessary suffering, sometimes lasting as many as fifty years. Before that diagnostic methodology could be developed, however, the symptoms of the underlying dissociative condition had to be understood. While eminent

---

[3]For studies relevant to dissociation in trauma survivors, see Carlson, Dalenberg, and McDade-Montez 2012; Lyssenko, Schmahl, and Bockhacker 2018; Spiegel and Cardena 1990; Wolf, Lunney, Miller et al. 2012.

theorists such as Janet and Prince explored dissociation in case studies more than a century old (Janet 1907; Prince 1925), only over the last thirty-five years have the basic components of this ubiquitous defense mechanism been examined systematically and clarified on the basis of large-scale, replicable investigations. Until then, lack of empirical research led some psychiatrists to wonder whether dissociative identity disorder, the most complex of those disorders, was a genuine condition, or even iatrogenic (Brand, Sar, Stavropoulos et al. 2016; Loewenstein 2018). And when doctors did accept the disorder's reality, diagnostic methods varied in sensitivity, with missed cases of dissociative identity disorder risking decompensation due to the lack of trauma-informed treatment.

I still remember, when I was in training, witnessing a woman named Gloria in the psychiatric inpatient unit receive sodium amobarbital (Amytal), a sedative meant to allow her alternate personalities to emerge, which, if present, would facilitate diagnosis of what was then known as Multiple Personality Disorder. Before our eyes, Gloria switched to a tearful adolescent alter who complained in a high, girlish voice about the hopelessness of her life. Suddenly she switched to an even more childish alter who babbled about the "bad booboos that Mommy and Daddy did." There was no doubt that Gloria was suffering from a dissociative disorder and needed treatment. But later, when I asked about her, I learned that she'd fled the hospital the next day after the Amytal had made her alters surface before a group of wide-eyed residents—including me. Humiliated, Gloria had bolted. I could understand why. Regret for the insensitivity she had suffered under the rubric of "training" turned this into a defining moment for me.

When I made it my mission to study dissociation, however, I encountered resistance. After completing my residency, I went to see a well-respected expert in psychiatry to inquire about my research options. As I told him about my plan to study dissociation, he listened with an inscrutable expression. I finished, and he cocked an eyebrow at me quizzically. He paused for a long moment. Then he said, as tactfully as he could, "Marlene, I would advise you that if you're interested in a successful career in research, find another subject."

Nevertheless, I persisted. Four years later, in 1989, I was awarded the first of two substantial grants from the National Institute of Mental Health, the first ever given to a researcher in dissociation. These grants allowed me to further refine my Five Component Model for Dissociation Assessment and conduct field trials of the Structured Clinical Interview for DSM-III-R Dissociative Disorders—the SCID-D, for short—the specialized interview I'd developed to meet the need for reliable dissociative symptom and disorder diagnosis. Over the course of the field trials, over three hundred interviews were conducted by ten clinicians, producing over one thousand hours of videotaped interviews. Those tapes were then reviewed; the data were analyzed to identify and validate the salient features that distinguished those who were suffering from a dissociative disorder from those who weren't. When we studied the results, it became clear that the clinicians' independent assessments almost always agreed, establishing high inter-rater reliability for the SCID-D. Finally, in 1993, the SCID-D and *Interviewer's Guide* were published for widespread use (Steinberg 1993a, 1993b). Since then, the interview has been administered with adolescents as young as eleven, and adults, in French, German, Hebrew, Korean, Turkish, Dutch, Norwegian, Spanish, Filipino, Danish, Persian, and more. Decades of international research and clinical experience have replicated our findings and established the SCID-D's reputation as the "gold standard" of dissociation assessment (Aquarone 2022; Boon and Draijer 1991, 1993; Carrion and Steiner 2000; Chang, Chang, Shiah, and Huang 2005; Friedl and Draijer 2000; Gast, Rodewald, and Nickel 2001; Gingrich 2004; Jepsen, Langeland, Sexton et al. 2014; Kim, Kim, and Jung 2016; Knudsen, Draijer, Haselrud, et al. 1995; Kundakçi, Sar, Kiziltan et al. 2014; Mohajerin, Lynn, Bakhtiyari et al. 2020; Mueller-Pfeiffer, Rufibach, and Wyss 2013; Mychailyszyn, Brand, Webermann et al. 2020; Piedfort-Marin, Tarquinio, Steinberg et al. 2021; Rodewald 2005; Sar, Onder, Kilicaslan et al. 2014; Steinberg 1995, 2000; Steinberg and Steinberg 1995; Steinberg, Cicchetti, Buchanan et al. 1994; Steinberg, Rounsaville, and Cicchetti 1990, 1991; Welburn, Fraser, Jordan et al. 2003).

Although theoretical models of dissociation existed, a practical model for clinical assessment was lacking. The SCID-D implements the Five Component Model of Dissociation Assessment and fills this need. As I define it for the purpose of clinical assessment, dissociation can be characterized by five primary components: **amnesia, depersonalization, derealization, identity confusion,** and **identity alteration.**[4] While I created the following definitions for "amnesia," "identity confusion," and "identity alteration," the definitions for "depersonalization" and "derealization" were synthesized from the literature.

- *Amnesia* refers to a subjective sense of gaps in one's memory for autobiographical information or experiences, or for blocks of time that have passed, where such lapses cannot be attributed to ordinary forgetfulness.

- *Depersonalization* refers to a feeling of disconnection from oneself (e.g., from one's feelings, thoughts, behavior, or body), or a sense of being an outside observer of one's self.

- *Derealization* refers to a feeling of disconnection from one's surroundings (e.g., people or surroundings feel as if they are unfamiliar, unreal, or distorted).

- *Identity confusion* refers to subjective feelings of uncertainty, puzzlement, conflict, or struggle regarding one's own identity or sense of self.

- *Identity alteration* refers to observable behavior associated with alterations or shifts in one's identity or personality states.

---

[4]Though the terms "symptom" and "component" may appear to be used interchangeably throughout the text, there is a subtle distinction. Recently, I introduced the term "component" to depathologize each dissociative experience— amnesia, depersonalization, derealization, identity confusion, and identity alteration—associated with dissociation. Additionally, I use the term to emphasize that such behaviors occur along a spectrum of severity, defined by the SCID-D assessment model's severity rating definitions. Dissociative behaviors that cause distress or compromise functioning are labeled "symptomatic," since the term connotes illness or a condition. Behaviors that don't compromise functioning or cause distress are referred to more neutrally as "components."

Identifying the five primary components of dissociation, developing their standard definitions, and using a standardized method to rate their severity are three major innovations in the SCID-D's assessment of dissociation.

In what sense are these components primary? Just as all other colors can be obtained by mixing the primary colors—red, yellow, and blue—so all posttraumatic dissociative experiences can be understood as consisting of a mixture of these five components. As with a primary color, the intensity of each component varies along a spectrum. On the one end, each can be a normative, transient coping mechanism that does not cause dysfunction or distress. On the other end, each can be recurrent or ongoing, interfering with relationships, causing internal suffering, or otherwise impairing functioning.

Consider flashbacks, a common dissociative experience. What mixture of these components constitutes a flashback? People who experience traumatic flashbacks, including rape survivors and veterans with PTSD, at the time feel disconnected from their current surroundings (derealization), behave as they would have at the time of the trauma (identity alteration), and have memory lapses for events happening around them in the present (amnesia). Another common dissociative behavior is sleepwalking. An individual who sleepwalks has no recollection of their sleepwalking activities (amnesia) and may behave very differently from how they usually would (identity alteration). All other dissociative experiences can be composed in this way using the five primary components as building blocks. Similarly, specific dissociative *disorders* can also be characterized by their various combinations of the five components—for instance, a moderate-to-severe level of amnesia with none-to-mild levels of the other four symptoms characterizes a diagnosis of Dissociative Amnesia, whereas moderate-to-severe levels of four or five components characterize Dissociative Identity Disorder.

Too frequently, systematic assessment for dissociative processes is overlooked, and the external signs of dissociation (e.g., intrusive thoughts, mood swings, somatization) are not linked to underlying dissociative conditions. The failure to detect dissociation can lead to ineffective treatment, higher rates of hospitalization and suicide attempts, and generally prolonged suffering ((Brand, Classen, McNary et al. 2009; Foote, Smolin, and Neft 2008; Kluft 1985, 1987; Mueller, Moergeli, Assaloni et al. 2007; Mueller-Pfeiffer, Rufibach, Perron et al. 2012; Sar, Koyuncu, Ozturk et al. 2007; Tanner, Wyss, Perron et al. 2017; Zoroglu, Tuzun, and Sar 2003). The SCID-D allows clinicians to uncover this connection. By inquiring about the core components of dissociation, the interview gathers the information necessary to look beyond the outermost signs—like depression, anxiety, mood swings, and flashbacks—to establish whether the underlying ailment is dissociative. Like the radiologist's X-ray, the SCID-D reveals the internal structure of dissociation, thereby suggesting a roadmap for effective dissociation-informed treatment.

In the decades since the SCID-D was first published, research has established the interview's diagnostic accuracy across diverse cultures; the five components present universally in trauma survivors. Numerous investigators have also confirmed the SCID-D's good-to-excellent inter-rater reliability and discriminant validity (Boon and Draijer 1991, 1993; Chang, Chang, Shiah et al. 2005; Friedl and Draijer 2000; Gingrich 2004; Jepsen, Langeland, Sexton et al. 2014; Kim, Kim, and Jung 2016; Knudsen, Draijer, Haselrud, et al. 1995; Kundakçi, Sar, Kiziltan et al. 2014; Mohajerin, Lynn, Bakhtiyari et al. 2020; Piedfort-Marin, Tarquinio, Steinberg et al. 2021; Rodewald 2005; Sar, Onder, Kilicaslan et al. 2014; Steinberg 1995, 2000; Steinberg, Cicchetti, and Buchanan 1994; Steinberg, Rounsaville, and Cicchetti 1990, 1991; Welburn, Fraser, Jordan et al. 2003). A recent meta-analysis of fifteen studies overwhelmingly confirmed the interview's ability to identify individuals with dissociative disorders and distinguish them from other psychiatric disorders and controls (Mychailyszn, Brand, Weberman et al. 2020).

Furthermore, neuroimaging studies have confirmed that people diagnosed with Dissociative Identity Disorder (DID) using the SCID-D interview exhibit unique physiological reactions and cerebral blood flow patterns during identity shifts compared with control subjects, high fantasizers, or actors asked to simulate a shift (Reinders, Willemsen, Vos et al. 2012). These results demonstrate that DID is neither fantasy proneness nor role playing; the brain images simply cannot be simulated. Few diagnostic interviews in psychiatry have demonstrated such diagnostically discriminating findings confirmed by brain imaging studies.

Over the last twenty years, a growing number of studies have also investigated the neuroimaging biomarkers of dissociative disorders. Though findings have not always been consistent, studies of SCID-D-identified individuals with DID suggest that the indicators of dissociation include decreased volume in key brain regions related to memory and executive functioning, similar to the brain patterns displayed by those diagnosed with PTSD (Chalavi, Vissia, Giesen et al. 2015; Logue, van Rooij, Dennis et al. 2018; Roydeva and Reinders 2020). Furthermore, smaller hippocampal volumes were found to be significantly correlated with severe childhood trauma, as well as with increased dissociative symptoms in DID and PTSD (Chalavi, Vissia, Giesen et al. 2015; Dimitrova, Dean, Schlumpf et al. 2021). Research remains to be done to characterize the biomarkers associated with PTSD, its dissociative subtypes, and dissociative disorders generally—but all in all, over two hundred recent investigations have laid the groundwork for understanding the neuroscience of dissociation (Roydeva and Reinders 2020).

When I was developing the SCID-D, my intention was to make visible the hidden components of dissociation. By devising a practical framework and systematic method of inquiry, I hoped to enable detailed assessment of a person's inner world of dissociative experiences and provide clients and therapists with a language for symptoms previously unspoken. That was my original mission. Now, over three decades of use have revealed that, besides serving as a powerful assessment tool, the SCID-D also provides therapeutic benefits (Fisher 2017; Finn and Martin 2013; Finn, Fischer, and Handler 2012; Kluft 2015; Steinberg and Hall 1997). Unlike many psychological tests whose main goal is to gather diagnostic information, the SCID-D poses open-ended questions designed to elicit rich, clinically meaningful information about an individual's subjective sense of their experiences. The chance to discuss, in a nonjudgemental setting, previously hidden or misunderstood experiences can enhance the therapeutic alliance and promote valuable insights. Making space for the individual to develop a more coherent narrative about their dissociative experiences constitutes one of the interview's principal benefits. Lastly, it should be noted that the SCID-D offers therapeutic benefits precisely because it does not pathologize these normal human experiences. For this reason, the information elicited during the interview can be used during feedback and in therapy to validate, educate, and empower.

Since the SCID-D's first use in 1983, it's been gratifying to see increased interest and advances in the field of dissociation. Mental health professionals in specialty clinics, private practices, and forensic settings have used the interview for systematic assessment and client education and as a practical method of inquiry that can enhance treatment. And researchers worldwide have used it to study dissociation and its impact among all posttraumatic conditions, about which we still have so much to learn. This revised edition, informed by over thirty-five years of research and clinical experience, incorporates the following updates:

1. The title has been changed to *The SCID-D Interview: Dissociation Assessment in Therapy, Forensics, and Research* to highlight, in addition to its diagnostic value, the tool's therapeutic, forensic, and research applications.

    a. Reference to the DSM has been removed from the title to underscore that the SCID-D's assessment model does not depend on DSM or ICD nosology. The results of the SCID-D form a superset of information which can be mapped into the diagnostic criteria of any edition of the DSM or ICD.

    b. The acronym "SCID-D" has been updated and now stands for the "Semi-Structured Clinical Interview for Dissociative Symptoms and Disorders." This is intended to emphasize that in addition to the dissociative disorders, the interview can be used in identifying dissociative symptoms present in other psychiatric conditions.

2. The design has been streamlined for ease of use in clinical settings.

3. An expanded "Psychiatric and Medical History" section includes questions related to somatic symptoms for scoring based on ICD-11 (International Classification of Diseases, 11th Revision), the global standard for diagnosis. An optional follow-up section has also been added for exploring the new ICD classification of Partial DID. This new follow-up section may be useful for researchers investigating whether Partial DID is meaningfully distinct from DID.

4. For those new to the SCID-D, further instructions and optional questions have been included that guide the interviewer in exploring varied manifestations of dissociative symptoms. For those clinicians using the SCID-D as an adjunct to therapy, optional therapeutically relevant questions have been added to the Follow-Up sections of the interview.

The 2023 edition of the *Interviewer's Guide to the SCID-D*, which is under development and forthcoming from American Psychiatric Association Publishing, includes expanded information about feedback and psychoeducation based on interview results; applications of the SCID-D method in therapy; dissociation in varied psychiatric conditions (e.g., posttraumatic stress, psychotic, mood, and other anxiety conditions); use in adolescent, adult, and forensic populations; and SCID-D psychometrics. Cross-cultural manifestations of dissociation and updated scientific references have also been included.

The content and sequence of the original questions remain unchanged from previous editions. Assessment of the five components of dissociation along a spectrum forms the basis for identifying symptom severity. Open-ended questions still encourage personalized follow-up. And emphasis remains on the importance of bringing attuned interviewing skills to systematic inquiry. Since it was unnecessary to make major revisions to the interview itself, the good-to-excellent psychometric properties of the previous editions persist (Piedfort-Marin, Tarquinio, Steinberg et al. 2021).

If you're a clinician, I hope you will familiarize yourself with the interview, as well as the *Interviewer's Guide*. You might begin by weaving some of the questions into your assessments and therapy. If you find that a client suffers from dissociative experiences, consider setting aside time to administer the full interview. For specialized training, consider attending a workshop or scheduling supervision with an expert in dissociation.

In my own work, I've marveled at the effect the interview can have on people whose symptoms were once labelled treatment-resistant or "psychotic." When they hear their experience reflected back to them for the first time without judgment or misattribution, I watch hope return as fear dissolves. Gradually, they grant me their trust, and we begin to explore the hidden, internal world that holds, somewhere inside it, the key to healing. Often, the interview is the first step on the road to recovery for those suffering from posttraumatic dissociation—it's the beginning of a journey that, when all is said and done, may be the most meaningful journey a person takes in their lifetime. I hope you find this enhanced version of the SCID-D useful both as a diagnostic interview and as a therapeutic method for helping your clients lead more authentic, fulfilling lives.

REFERENCES

American Psychiatric Association: *Diagnostic and Statistical Manual of Mental Disorders*, 5th Edition. Arlington, VA, American Psychiatric Association, 2013

Bailey T., Boyer S., Brand B.: Dissociative disorders, in *Diagnostic Interviewing*. Edited by Segal D. New York, Springer, 2019, pp. 401–424

Bakim B., Baran E., Diyaddin M., et al.: Comparison of the patient groups with and without dissociative disorder comorbidity among the inpatients with bipolar disorder. *Family Practice & Palliative Care* 1(2):35-42, 2016

Boon S., Draijer N.: Diagnosing dissociative disorders in the Netherlands: a pilot study with the Structured Clinical Interview for DSM-III-R Dissociative Disorders. *American Journal of Psychiatry* 148:458–462, 1991

Boon S., Draijer N.: *Multiple Personality Disorder in the Netherlands: A Study on Reliability and Validity of the Diagnosis*. Lisse, the Netherlands, Swets & Zeitlinger Publishers, 1993

Bowman E.S.: Why conversion seizures should be classified as a dissociative disorder. *Psychiatric Clinics of North America* 29(1):185–211, 2006

Brand B.L., Loewenstein R., Spiegel D.: Dispelling myths about dissociative identity disorder treatment: an empirically based approach. *Psychiatry* 77(2):169–189, 2014

Brand B.L., Sar V., Stavropoulos P., et al.: Separating fact from fiction: an empirical examination of six myths about dissociative identity disorder. *Harvard Review of Psychiatry* 24(4):257–270, 2016

Brand B.L., Classen C.C., McNary S.W., Zaveri P.: A review of dissociative disorders treatment studies. *Journal of Nervous and Mental Disease* 197(9):646–654, 2009

Brand B.L., McNary S.W., Myrick A.C., et al.: A longitudinal naturalistic study of patients with dissociative disorders treated by community clinicians. *Psychological Trauma: Theory, Research, Practice, and Policy*, 5(4):301–308, 2013

Bremner D., Steinberg M., Southwick S., et al.: Use of the Structured Clinical Interview for DSM-IV Dissociative Disorders for systematic assessment of dissociative symptoms in posttraumatic stress disorder. *American Journal of Psychiatry* 150(7):1011–1014, 1993

Brown D., and Elliot D.: *Attachment Disturbances in Adults: Treatment for Comprehensive Repair*. New York, W.W. Norton, 2016

Carlson E., Dalenberg C., McDade-Montez E.: Dissociation in Posttraumatic Stress Disorder, Part I: definitions and review of research. *Psychological Trauma: Theory, Research, Practice, and Policy* 4(5):479–489, 2012

Carrion V., Steiner H.: Trauma and dissociation in delinquent adolescents. *Journal of the American Academy of Child and Adolescent Psychiatry* 39:353–359, 2000

Child and Adolescent Health Measurement Initiative: National Survey of Children's Health: Survey Year 2017–2018

Chalavi S., Vissia E.,Giesen M., et al.: Abnormal hippocampal morphology in dissociative identity disorder and post-traumatic stress disorder correlates with childhood trauma and dissociative symptoms. *Human Brain Mapping* 36(5):1692–1704, 2015

Chang A.J., Chang S.H., Shiah I.S., Huang C.W.: Preliminary study of the DES and SCID-D Chinese versions on college students of National Defense Medical Center. Paper presented at the the 22nd International Society for the Study of Dissociation International Conference, November 2005

Coons P.: The differential diagnosis of multiple personality. A comprehensive review. *Psychiatric Clinics of North America* 7(1):51–68, 1984

Coons P., Bowman E., Milstein V.: Multiple personality: a clinical investigation of 50 cases. *Journal of Nervous and Mental Disease* 176(9):519–527, 1988

Darvos-Bornoz J.: Rape-related psychotraumatic syndromes. *European Journal of Obstetrics & Gynecology and Reproductive Biology* 71(1):59–65, 1997

Darves-Bornoz J.M., Degiovanni A., Gaillard P.: Why is dissociative identity disorder infrequent in France. *American Journal of Psychiatry* 152(10):1530–1531, 1995

Darves-Bornoz J.M., Lépine J.P., Choquet M., et al.: Predictive factors of chronic post-traumatic stress disorder in rape victims. *European Psychiatry* 13(6):281–287, 1998

Darvos-Bornoz J., Berger C., Degiovanni A., et al.: Similarities and differences between incestuous and nonincestuous rape in a French follow-up study, *Journal of Traumatic Stress* 12(4):613–623, 1999

Dimitrova L.I., Dean S.L., Schlumpf Y.R. et al.: A neurostructural biomarker of dissociative amnesia: a hippocampal study in dissociative identity disorder. *Psychological Medicine* June 24; 1–9, 2021

Dorahy M., Van der Hart O.: DSM–5's Posttraumatic Stress Disorder with Dissociative Symptoms: challenges and future directions. *Journal of Trauma & Dissociation* 16:7–28, 2015

Fine C.: A cognitively based treatment model for DSM-IV dissociative identity disorder, in *Handbook of Dissociation*. Edited by Michelson L.K., Ray W.J. Boston, MA, Springer, 1996, pp. 401–441

Finn S., Martin H.: Therapeutic assessment: using psychological testing as brief therapy, in *APA Handbook of Testing and Assessment in Psychology, Vol. 2: Testing and Assessment in Clinical and Counseling Psychology*. Edited by Geisinger K.F., Bracken B.A., Carlson J.F., et al. Washington, DC, American Psychological Association, 2013, pp. 453–465

Finn S., Fischer C., Handler L. (eds.): *Collaborative/Therapeutic Assessment: A Casebook and Guide*. Hoboken, NJ, Wiley, 2012

Fisher J.: *Healing the Fragmented Selves of Trauma Survivors: Overcoming Internal Self-Alienation*. New York, Routledge, 2017

Foote B., Smolin Y., Neft D., et al.: Dissociative disorders and suicidality in psychiatric outpatients. *Journal of Nervous and Mental Disease* 196(1):29–36, 2008

Friedl M., Draijer N.: Dissociative disorders in Dutch psychiatric inpatients, *American Journal of Psychiatry* 157(6):1012–1013, 2000

Gast U., Rodewald F., Nickel V., et al.: Prevalence of dissociative disorders among psychiatric inpatients in a German university clinic. *Journal of Nervous and Mental Disease* 189:249–257, 2001

Gilbert P.: *Compassion Focused Therapy: Distinctive Features*. New York, Routledge, 2010

Gingrich H.: Dissociative symptoms in Filipino college students. *Philippine Journal of Psychology* 37(2):50–78, 2004

Goff D., Olin J., Jenike M., et al.: Dissociative symptoms in patients with obsessive-compulsive disorder. *Journal of Nervous and Mental Disease* 180(5):332–337, 1992

Haugen M., Castillo R.: Unrecognized dissociation in psychotic outpatients and implications of ethnicity. *Journal of Nervous and Mental Disease* 187(12):751–754, 1999

Herman J.: *Trauma and Recovery*. New York, Basic Books, 2015

Hill S., Wolff J., Bigony C., et al.: Dissociative subtype of posttraumatic stress disorder in women in partial and residential levels of psychiatric care. *Journal of Trauma & Dissociation* 21(3):305–318, 2019

Howell E.: *Trauma and Dissociation Informed Psychotherapy: Relational Healing and the Therapeutic Connection*. New York, W.W. Norton, 2020

International Society for the Study of Trauma and Dissociation: Guidelines for treating dissociative identity disorder in adults. *Journal of Trauma & Dissociation* 6(4):69–149, 2005

Janet P.: *The Major Symptoms of Hysteria: Fifteen Lectures Given in the Medical School of Harvard University*. New York, Macmillan, 1907

Jepsen E., Langeland W., Sexton H., et al.: Inpatient treatment for early sexually abused adults: a naturalistic 12-month follow-up study. *Psychological Trauma: Theory, Research, Practice, and Policy* 6(2):142–151, 2014

Johnson J., Cohen P., Kasen S., Brook J.: Dissociative disorders among adults in the community, impaired functioning, and axis I and II comorbidity. *Journal of Psychiatric Research* 40(2):131–140, 2006

Karadag F., Sar V., Tamar-Gurol D., et al.: Dissociative disorders among inpatients with drug or alcohol dependency. *Journal of Clinical Psychiatry* 66(10):1247–1253, 2005

Kim I., Kim D., Jung H.: Dissociative identity disorders in Korea: two recent cases. Psychiatry Investigation 13(2):250–252, 2016

Kluft R.: The natural history of multiple personality disorder, in *Childhood Antecedents of Multiple Personality*. Edited by Kluft R.P. Washington, DC, American Psychiatric Press, 1985, pp. 197–238

Kluft R.: First-rank symptoms as a diagnostic clue to multiple personality disorder. *American Journal of Psychiatry* 144(3):293–298, 1987

Kluft R.: Basic principles in conducting the psychotherapy of multiple personality disorder, in *Clinical Perspectives on Multiple Personality Disorder*. Edited by Kluft R.P., Fine C.G. Washington, DC, American Psychiatric Press, 1993, pp. 19–50

Kluft R.: A clinician's understanding of dissociation: fragments of an acquaintance, in Dissociation and the Dissociative Disorders. Edited by O'Neil J., Dell P. New York, Routledge, 2015, pp. 599–624

Kluft R., Bloom S., Kinzie J.: Treating the traumatized patient and victims of violence. *New Directions in Mental Health Services* Summer (86)79–102, 2000

Knudsen, H., Draijer, N., Haselrud, J., Boe, T., et al.: Dissociative disorders in Norwegian psychiatric inpatients. Paper presented at the Spring meeting of the International Society for the Study of Dissociation, Amsterdam, The Netherlands, 1995

Kundakçi T., Sar V., Kiziltan E., et al.: Reliability and validity of the Turkish version of the Structured Clinical Interview for DSM-IV Dissociative Disorders (SCID-D): a preliminary study. *Journal of Trauma & Dissociation* 15(1):24–34, 2014

Loewenstein R.J.: Dissociation debates: everything you know is wrong. *Dialogues in Clinical Neuroscience* 20(3):229–242, 2018

Logue M.W., van Rooij S.J.H., Dennis E.L., et al.: Smaller hippocampal volume in posttraumatic stress disorder: a multisite ENIGMA-PGC study: subcortical volumetry results from posttraumatic stress disorder consortia. *Biological Psychiatry* 83(3):244–253, 2018

Lyssenko L., Schmahl C., Bockhacker L., et al.: Dissociation in psychiatric disorders: a meta-analysis of studies using the dissociative experiences scale. *American Journal of Psychiatry* 175(1):37–46, 2018

Mohajerin B., Lynn S., Bakhtiyari M., et al.: Evaluating the unified protocol in the treatment of dissociative identify disorder. *Cognitive and Behavioral Practice* 27(3):270–289, 2020

Mueller C., Moergeli H., Assaloni H., et.al.: Dissociative disorders among chronic and severely impaired psychiatric outpatients. *Psychopathology* 40(6):470–471, 2007

Mueller-Pfeiffer C., Rufibach K., Perron N., et al.: Global functioning and disability in dissociative disorders. *Psychiatry Research* 200(2–3):475–481, 2012

Mueller-Pfeiffer C., Rufibach K., Wyss D., et al.: Screening for dissociative disorders in psychiatric out- and day care–patients. *Journal of Psychopathology and Behavioral Assessment* 35(4):592–602, 2013

Mychailyszyn M., Brand B., Webermann A., et al.: Differentiating dissociative from non-dissociative disorders: a meta-analysis of the structured clinical interview for DSM dissociative disorders (SCID-D). *Journal of Trauma & Dissociation* 22(1):1–16, 2020

Nijenhuis E.: Somatoform dissociation: major symptoms of dissociative disorders. *Journal of Trauma & Dissociation* 1(4):7–32, 2000

Perry B., Dobson C.: The neurosequential model of therapeutics, in *Treating Complex Traumatic Stress Disorders in Children and Adolescents: Scientific Foundations and Therapeutic Models*. Edited by Ford J., Courtois C. New York, Guilford Press, 2013, pp. 249–260

Piedfort-Marin O., Tarquinio C., Steinberg M., et al.: Reliability and validity study of the French-language version of the SCID-D semi-structured clinical interview for diagnosing DSM-5 and ICD-11 dissociative disorders. *Annales Médico-psychologiques* 180(6):51–59, 2022

Prince M.: *The Dissociation of a Personality*. London, Longmans, Green, & Co., 1925

Putnam F., Guroff J., Silberman E.K., et al.: The clinical phenomenology of multiple personality disorder: review of 100 recent cases. *Journal of Clinical Psychiatry* 47(6):285–293, 1986

Reinders A.A.T.S., Willemsen A.T.M., Vos H.P.J., et al.: Fact or factitious? A psychobiological study of authentic and simulated dissociative identity states. *PloS One* 7(6), 2012

Roco V., Hart J., Kinbrell T., et al.: Cognitive function and dissociative disorder status among veteran subjects with chronic posttraumatic stress disorder: a preliminary study. *Journal of Neuropsychiatry and Clinical Neurosciences* 18(2):226–230, 2006

Rodewald F.: Diagnostics of dissociative disorders. Doctoral dissertation, Hannover Medical School, Hanover, Germany, 2005

Roydeva MI, Reinders AATS: Biomarkers of pathological dissociation: a systematic review. *Neuroscience and Biobehavioral Reviews* 123(1):120–202, 2020

Sar V.: Epidemiology of dissociative disorders: an overview. *Epidemiology Research International* 404538, 2011

Sar V., Onder C., Kilicaslan A., et al.: Dissociative identity disorder among adolescents: prevalence in a university psychiatric outpatient unit. *Journal of Trauma & Dissociation* 15(4):402–419, 2014

Sar V., Kundakci T., Kiziltan E., et al.: The axis-I dissociative disorder comorbidity of borderline personality disorder among psychiatric outpatients. *Journal of Trauma & Dissociation* 4(1):119–136, 2003

Sar V., Koyuncu A., Ozturk E., et al.: Dissociative disorders in the psychiatric emergency ward. *General Hospital Psychiatry* 29(1):45–50, 2007

Schwartz R.: *Introduction to the Internal Family Systems*. Oak Park, IL, Trailheads Publications, 2001

Siegel D: *The Developing Mind, How Relationships and the Brain Interact to Shape Who We Are*. New York, Guilford Press, 2020

Sinason V (ed.): *Attachment, Trauma, and Multiplicity*. East Sussex, UK, Routledge, 2010

Somer E., Altusa L., Ginzburg K.: Dissociative psychopathology among opioid use disorder patients: exploring the "chemical dissociation" hypothesis. *Comprehensive Psychiatry* 51:419–425, 2010

Spiegel D., Cardena E.: Dissociative mechanisms in posttraumatic stress disorder, in *Posttraumatic Stress Disorder: Etiology, Phenomenology, and Treatment*. Edited by Wolf M., Mosnaim A. Washington, DC, American Psychiatric Press, 1990, pp. 23–34

Spiegel D., Rosenfeld A.A.: Spontaneous hypnotic age regression: case report. *Journal of Clinical Psychiatry* 45(12):522–524, 1984

Steele K., Van der Hart O., Nijenhuis E.: Phase-oriented treatment of structural dissociation in complex traumatization: overcoming trauma related phobias. *Journal of Trauma & Dissociation* 6(3):11–53, 2005

Steinberg M.: *Interviewer's Guide to the Structured Clinical Interview for DSM-IV Dissociative Disorders (SCID-D).* Washington, DC, American Psychiatric Press, 1993a

Steinberg M.: *Structured Clinical Interview for DSM-IV-R Dissociative Disorders (SCID-D).* Washington, DC, American Psychiatric Press, 1993b

Steinberg M.: *Handbook for the Assessment of Dissociation: A Clinical Guide.* Washington, DC, American Psychiatric Press, 1995

Steinberg M.: Advances in the clinical assessment of dissociation: the SCID-D-R. *Bulletin of the Menninger Clinic* 64(2):146–163, 2000 Available at: https://www.researchgate.net/profile/ Marlene-Steinberg/publication/12476744_Advances_in_the_clinical_assessment_ of_dissociation_The_SCID-D-R/links/54832b300cf2f5dd63a90fcd/ Advances-in-the-clinical-assessment-of-dissociation-The-SCID-D-R.pdf.

Steinberg M., Schnall M.: *The Stranger in the Mirror: Dissociation—The Hidden Epidemic.* New York, HarperCollins, 2010

Steinberg M., Steinberg A.: Systematic assessment of dissociative identity disorder in adolescents using the SCID-D: three case studies. *Bulletin of the Menninger Clinic* 59:221–231, 1995

Steinberg M., Hall P.: The SCID-D diagnostic interview and treatment planning in dissociative disorders. *Bulletin of the Menninger Clinic* 61:108–120, 1997

Steinberg M., Cicchetti D., Buchanan J., et al.: Distinguishing between multiple personality disorder and schizophrenia using the structured clinical interview for DSM-IV dissociative disorders (SCID-D). *Journal of Nervous and Mental Disease* 182(9):495–502, 1994

Steinberg M., Rounsaville B.J., Cicchetti D.V.: The structured clinical interview for DSM-III-R dissociative disorders: preliminary report on a new diagnostic instrument. *American Journal of Psychiatry* 147(1):76–82, 1990

Steinberg M., Rounsaville B.J., Cicchetti D.V.: Detection of dissociative disorders in psychiatric patients by a screening instrument and a structured diagnostic interview. *American Journal of Psychiatry* 148(8):1050–1054, 1991

Steinberg M., Barry D., Sholomskas D., and Hall P.: SCL-90 symptom patterns: indicators of dissociative disorders. *Bulletin of the Menninger Clinic* 69(3):237–249, 2005

Swart S., Wildschut M., Draijer N., et al.: Dissociative subtype of posttraumatic stress disorder or PTSD with comorbid dissociative disorders: comparative evaluation of clinical profiles. *Psychological Trauma: Theory, Research, Practice and Policy* 12(1):38–45, 2020

Tanner J., Wyss D., Perron N., et al.: Frequency and characteristics of suicide attempts in dissociative identity disorders: a 12-month follow-up study in psychiatric outpatients in Switzerland. *European Journal of Trauma & Dissociation* 1(4):235–239, 2017

Van der Hart O., Nijenhuis E., Steele K.: Dissociation: an insufficiently recognized major feature of complex posttraumatic stress disorder. *Journal of Traumatic Stress* 18(5):413–424, 2005

Van der Hart O., Nijenhuis E., Steele K.: *The Haunted Self: Structural Dissociation and the Treatment of Chronic Traumatization*. New York, W.W. Norton, 2006

Watkins H., Watkins J.: *Ego States: Theory and Therapy*. New York, W.W. Norton, 1997

Welburn K.R., Fraser G.A., Jordan S.A., et al.: Discriminating dissociative identity disorder from schizophrenia and feigned dissociation on psychological tests and structured interviews. *Journal of Trauma & Dissociation* 4(2):109–130, 2003

Wolf E., Lunney C., Miller M., et al.: The dissociative subtype of PTSD: a replication and extension. *Depression and Anxiety* 29(8):679–688, 2012

Zoroglu S., Tuzun U., Sar V.: Suicide attempt and self-mutilation among Turkish high school students in relation with abuse, neglect and dissociation. *Psychiatry and Clinical Neurosciences* 57(1):119–126 2003

xxiv

PART I:
PSYCHIATRIC AND MEDICAL HISTORY

History Questions

This SCID-D interview allows for systematic assessment of dissociative symptoms and disorders. This initial section asks about psychiatric and medical history and other background information that can help inform diagnosis. Note: Questions marked with an asterisk ("*") are optional for diagnostic purposes but may provide additional, clinically relevant information. Questions appearing in parenthesis are of two types: 1) optional rewordings of a SCID-D question or 2) examples of possible follow-up questions that the interviewer may wish to pursue. The interviewer is encouraged to ask their own follow-up questions in pursuit of clarification or elaboration of a client's response to SCID-D questions.

I'll start by asking you questions about your background and experiences you may have had. I'll be taking notes as we talk. Do you have any questions before we begin?	
Demographic Information	
H1. How old are you?	Age: _____
H2. Which gender do you identify with?	**Gender Identity** ◯ female ◯ male ◯ nonbinary ◯ other (please specify): _____ ◯ prefer not to say
H3. What is the highest level of education that you have completed?	**Education Level** ◯ graduate school ◯ college (4 year) ◯ college (2 year) or technical school ◯ high school ◯ did not complete high school
H4. What is your marital status?	**Marital Status** ◯ married ◯ living together with partner ◯ separated ◯ divorced/annulled ◯ widowed ◯ never married

Cite as: Steinberg M: The SCID-D Interview: Dissociation Assessment in Therapy, Forensics, and Research. Washington, DC, American Psychiatric Association Publishing, 2023

H5. With whom do you live?	Description:
H6. Do you have children? 　IF YES: How old are they?	**Children** ○ Unclear　○ No　○ Yes
Work History	
H7. Are you working? 　IF YES: What kind of work do you do? How long have you worked there? 　IF NO: What kind of work did you do in the past? (When was the last time you were employed?)	**Working Currently** ○ Unclear　○ No　○ Yes Description:
H8. What is the longest period of time you have been employed?	Description:
H9. Has there ever been a time when you were unable to work? 　IF YES: When was that? Why were you unable to work?	**Unable to Work** ○ Unclear　○ No　○ Yes Description:
Psychiatric History	
H10. Have you ever been in therapy (as an outpatient)? 　IF YES: What first led you to seek treatment? (How old were you? Approximately how many therapists have you worked with? When was the last time you were in therapy?)	**Outpatient Therapy** ○ Unclear　○ No　○ Yes Description:

H11. Are you currently being treated with medication for psychological problems? IF YES: What medication are you taking? Have you been treated with other psychiatric medication in the past? IF YES: What medications have you been treated with?	**Psychiatric Medication** ◯ Unclear ◯ No ◯ Yes Description:
H12. Have you ever been hospitalized for psychiatric treatment? IF YES: What led to your hospitalization and when did this occur?	**Psychiatric Hospitalization** ◯ Unclear ◯ No ◯ Yes Description:
H12a. How many times have you been hospitalized (for psychiatric treatment)? (What was the longest time that you were hospitalized?)	Description:
H13. Have you ever harmed yourself or thought about harming yourself (including cutting, burning, suicide attempts)? IF YES: Can you describe what occurred? (How old were you when you first tried to hurt yourself? Approximately how many times have you tried to hurt yourself?)	**Self-Harm** ◯ Unclear ◯ No ◯ Yes Description:

Alcohol Use History	
H14. During the past year, how often have you had a drink that contains alcohol?	**Frequency of Drinking (past year)** ○ unclear ○ 0 to 5 times in past year ○ 6 to 11 times in past year ○ 1 to 2 times per month ○ up to 3 times per month ○ 1 to 3 times a week ○ 4 to 7 times a week
H15. How many drinks do you usually have when you are drinking (during the past year)?	**Number of Drinks** ○ 2 or fewer ○ 3 or 4 ○ 5 or 6 ○ 7 or more
H16. Prior to the past year, how often did you have a drink that contained alcohol?	**Frequency of Drinking (prior to past year)** ○ unclear ○ 0 to 5 times per year ○ 6 to 11 times per year ○ 1 to 2 times per month ○ up to 3 times per month ○ 1 to 3 times a week ○ 4 to 7 times a week
H17. How many drinks did you usually have when you were drinking (prior to the past year)?	**Number of Drinks** ○ 2 or fewer ○ 3 or 4 ○ 5 or 6 ○ 7 or more
H18. Has drinking ever interfered with your relationships or your ability to function? IF YES: In what way did it interfere?	**Interfered with Relationships or Functioning** ○ Unclear ○ No ○ Yes Description:
If the client denies significant alcohol use, skip ahead to question H22 (Drug Use History, page 8). If the client endorses alcohol use, continue with H19.	

H19. When was the last time you had five or more drinks at one occasion?	**Drinking Five or More Drinks** ○ never ○ prior to past year ○ past year ○ past month ○ past week
H20. Have you ever had treatment for alcohol use?	**Treatment for Alcohol Use** ○ Unclear ○ No ○ Yes
IF NO treatment for alcohol use, skip to question H22 (Drug Use History, page 8). IF YES, continue with H20a.	
H20a. Did you have treatment as an out-patient? (When did you receive treatment?)	**Outpatient Alcohol Treatment** ○ Unclear ○ No ○ Yes
H20b. Were you ever hospitalized for treatment of your alcohol use? IF YES: **H20c.** How many times were you hospitalized? (When was the first time you were hospitalized for alcohol use? When was the last time you were hospitalized?)	**Inpatient Alcohol Treatment** ○ Unclear ○ No ○ Yes **Number of Hospitalizations for Alcohol Abuse** ○ 1–2 ○ 3–4 ○ 5–6 ○ 7 or more times Description:
H20d. Did you ever have residential treatment for alcohol use? (How many times have you been in residential treatment?)	**Residential Alcohol Treatment** ○ Unclear ○ No ○ Yes

H21. What is the longest period of time that you were able to avoid using any alcohol (be abstinent)?	**Longest Period of Abstinence From Alcohol** ◯ days ◯ weeks ◯ months ◯ 1 year–3 years ◯ more than 3 years–6 years ◯ more than 6 years
Drug Use History	
H22. Have you ever used prescription drugs in doses that were higher than prescribed or for longer periods of time? IF YES: What prescription drugs did you use? (When did you first begin to use ————? _(endorsed drug) How long did that last?)	**Prescription Drug Abuse** ◯ Unclear ◯ No ◯ Yes Description:
H23. Have you ever used drugs (other than those prescribed for medical reasons)?	**Drug Use** ◯ Unclear ◯ No ◯ Yes
IF NO to drug use, skip to question H27 (Medical History, page 10) IF YES, continue with question H24.	
H24. What drugs have you used? (Have you used any of the following drugs?)	Description:

	Drug Use		Age(s) Used
H24a. Marijuana	◯ No	◯ Yes	_____
H24b. Cocaine	◯ No	◯ Yes	_____
H24c. Heroin or other opioids	◯ No	◯ Yes	_____
H24d. Hallucinogens	◯ No	◯ Yes	_____
H24e. Amphetamines	◯ No	◯ Yes	_____
H24f. Pain medication	◯ No	◯ Yes	_____
H24g. Inhalants	◯ No	◯ Yes	_____
H24h. Other prescription medication: _____	◯ No	◯ Yes	_____
H24i. Other: _____	◯ No	◯ Yes	_____

H24j. How old were you when you first used _____? How old were you when you last used _____? (endorsed drug) *(Record ages on right side of questions H24a-i.)*	Description:
H24k. In the past month, have you used any drugs? IF YES: What drug did you use and how often? When was the last time you used _____? (endorsed drug)	**Drug Use During Past Month** ○ Unclear ○ No ○ Yes Description:
H25. Have you ever had treatment for drug use?	**Treatment for Drug Use** ○ Unclear ○ No ○ Yes
IF NO drug treatment, skip to question H27 (Medical History, page 10). IF YES, continue with H25a.	
H25a. Did you have treatment as an out-patient? (When did you receive treatment?)	**Outpatient Drug Treatment** ○ Unclear ○ No ○ Yes
H25b. Were you ever hospitalized for treatment of drug use? (When was the first time you were hospitalized for drug use? When was the last time you were hospitalized?)	**Inpatient Drug Treatment** ○ Unclear ○ No ○ Yes
IF YES: **H25c.** How many times were you hospitalized?	**Number of Hospitalizations for Drug Use** ○ 1–2 ○ 3–4 ○ 5–6 ○ 7 or more
H25d. Did you ever have residential treatment for drug use? (How many times have you been in residential treatment?)	**Residential Drug Treatment** ○ Unclear ○ No ○ Yes

H26. What is the longest period of time that you were able to avoid using any drugs (be abstinent)?	**Longest Period of Abstinence From Drugs** ○ days ○ weeks ○ months ○ 1 year–3 years ○ more than 3 years–6 years ○ more than 6 years
<u>**Medical History**</u> **Now I'll be asking you some questions about your medical history.**	
H27. Do you have any medical problems? IF YES: What medical problems do you have?	**Medical Problems** ○ Unclear ○ No ○ Yes Description:
H28. Are you being treated with medication for any medical problems? IF YES: What medication are you taking?	**Medication for Medical Illness** ○ Unclear ○ No ○ Yes Description:
H29. Have you ever experienced a serious side effect of a prescribed medication that led you to discontinue the medication? IF YES: What medication were you taking and what side effect did you experience? (How long did that side effect last? When did you experience that side effect?)	**Medication Side Effect** ○ Unclear ○ No ○ Yes Description:

H30. Have you ever been hospitalized for medical treatment? IF YES: What led to your hospitalization? How many times were you hospitalized? (How old were you when you were hospitalized?)	**Hospitalized for Medical Treatment** ○ Unclear ○ No ○ Yes Description:
H31. Have you ever had a head injury? IF YES: Can you describe what occurred? (How old were you when you had a head injury?)	**Head Injury** ○ Unclear ○ No ○ Yes Description:
H31a. Did you see a doctor? IF YES: What did the doctor say about your head injury?	**Consult a Doctor** ○ Unclear ○ No ○ Yes Description:
H31b. Did you experience loss of consciousness at the time of the head injury? IF YES: Can you describe what occurred?	**Loss of Consciousness With Head Injury** ○ Unclear ○ No ○ Yes Description:
H32. Have you ever had seizures that were diagnosed by a doctor or been told by someone who observed you having a seizure? IF YES: Can you describe what you experienced or were told? What type of seizure did the doctor (or someone you know) say you had? Did you have an EEG (electroencephalogram)? IF YES: Do you know the results of the EEG?	**Seizure History** ○ Unclear ○ No ○ Yes Description:
H32a. Were you treated with medication? IF YES: What medication? **H32b.** When was the first time you had a seizure? When was the last time you had a seizure? How often do/did you have seizures?	**Seizures Treated With Medication** ○ Unclear ○ No ○ Yes Description:

Family History (parents, siblings, other relatives)			
H33. Does anyone in your family have a history of psychiatric illness or alcohol or drug use?	**Family History: Psychiatric Illness**　　○ Unclear　　○ No　　○ Yes		
IF YES: What type of problems do/did they have? (Does any relative have any of the following problems?)	**Parent**	**Sibling**	**Other Relative**
H33a. Schizophrenia	○	○	○
H33b. Major Depression	○	○	○
H33c. Bipolar Disorder	○	○	○
H33d. Anxiety Disorder	○	○	○
H33e. Posttraumatic Stress Disorder	○	○	○
H33f. Dissociative Disorder	○	○	○
H33g. Alcohol Use Disorder	○	○	○
H33h. Drug Use Disorder	○	○	○
H33i. Undiagnosed Psychiatric Symptoms	○	○	○
H33j. Other	○	○	○

Imaginary Friend History	
H34. As a child did you ever have an imaginary friend(s)? IF YES: Can you describe the imaginary friend? How old were you when you had _____? (client's endorsed experience) How long was this imaginary friend a part of your life? (Can you remember having any conversations with _____? (client's endorsed experience) IF YES: Can you share an example of the conversations you had?)	**Imaginary Friend** ○ Unclear ○ No ○ Yes Description:
FOR ICD-11 DIAGNOSES: Continue with H35. *FOR DSM-5 DIAGNOSES: You may skip ahead to page 19 and continue with question 1 (Amnesia History). (Questions H35–H39 are not necessary for DSM diagnoses. However, if you are interested in exploring somatic symptoms, feel free to continue with H35.)*	
Pseudoseizures and **Other Somatic Symptoms History**	*(Dissociative processes commonly express somatically [e.g., changes in movement, sensation, or perception without medical origin]. For example, visual and perceptual distortions may occur in association with derealization in individuals with Depersonalization-Derealization Disorder.)*
H35. Have you ever experienced unwanted movements such as shaking, "seizure-like" movements, or loss of balance, without known medical cause? IF YES: What symptoms did you experience? How often has that occurred? (How long did _____ last? Did it interfere with (endorsed symptoms) your functioning?) IF YES: How did it interfere with your functioning?	**Pseudoseizures/Other Unwanted Movements** ○ Unclear ○ No ○ Yes Description:

H35a. Did you see a doctor?

IF YES: What did the doctor say about your symptoms?

IF YES to "seizure-like" movements, continue with H35b. IF NO, skip to H36.

Consult With a Doctor
O Unclear   O No   O Yes

Description:

H35b. Did you lose consciousness following

the ————————?
    (endorsed movements)

IF YES: Can you describe that experience? How often has that occurred? How long did it last?

Loss of Consciousness
O Unclear   O No   O Yes
(In dissociative nonepileptic seizures, there is typically no loss of consciousness.)

Description:

H35c. Did you experience any tongue-biting, serious bruising, cuts (due to falling), or urine loss (due to the "seizure-like" episodes)?

IF YES: What did you experience?

Tongue-biting, Cuts, Urinary Incontinence
O Unclear   O No   O Yes
(In dissociative nonepileptic seizures, there is typically no tongue-biting, serious bruising, cuts, or urine loss.)

Description:

H35d. Did you have an EEG (electroencephalogram)?
IF YES: What was the result of the EEG?

Had EEG
O Unclear   O No   O Yes

Description:

H35e. Were you (are you being) treated with any medication?

IF YES: What medication?

Use of Medication
O Unclear   O No   O Yes

Description:

H36. Have you ever experienced any visual problems or loss of vision such as visual snow, tunnel vision, or distorted vision (unrelated to eye disease or a medical condition)?

IF YES: Can you describe what you experienced? (How often has that occurred? How long did it last? Did it interfere with your functioning? IF YES: How did it interfere?)

H36a. Did you see a doctor?

IF YES: What did the doctor say was the cause of your visual problems?

Visual Problems (without medical cause)
○ Unclear   ○ No   ○ Yes

Description:

Consult With a Doctor
○ Unclear   ○ No   ○ Yes

Description:

H37. Have you ever lost or experienced changes in any of your senses (vision, hearing, touch, smell, vibration, pain, or ability to feel heat or cold) without known medical cause?

IF YES: What type of change or loss in senses did you experience? (How often has that occurred? How long did it last?)

H37a. Did you see a doctor?
IF YES: What did the doctor say was the cause of your change or loss of sensation?

Changes or Loss of Senses
○ Unclear   ○ No   ○ Yes

Description:

Consult With a Doctor
○ Unclear   ○ No   ○ Yes

Description:

H38. Have you ever experienced dizziness or vertigo that interfered with your functioning (without known medical cause)?

IF YES: What symptoms did you experience? (How often has that occurred? How long did it last? How did it interfere with your functioning?)

H38a. Did you see a doctor?

IF YES: What did the doctor say was the cause of your dizziness (or vertigo)?

Dizziness
○ Unclear   ○ No   ○ Yes

Description:

Consult With a Doctor
○ Unclear   ○ No   ○ Yes

Description:

H39. Have you ever experienced changes or a loss in your ability to speak, swallow, or move any part of your body (without known medical cause)?

  IF YES: What symptoms did you experience? (How often has that occurred? How long did it last? Did it interfere with your functioning?) IF YES: How did it interfere?

H39a. Did you see a doctor?

  IF YES: What did the doctor say was the cause of your symptoms?

Changes or Loss of Speech or Movement
O Unclear   O No   O Yes

Description:

Consult With a Doctor
O Unclear   O No   O Yes

Description:

PART II:
THE FIVE COMPONENTS OF
DISSOCIATION ASSESSMENT

AMNESIA:
PAST AND CURRENT SYMPTOMS

Sometimes memory can help us explore what a person's life is like. I'll start by asking you some questions about your memory.	*(For clinical assessment of dissociation, the author has defined amnesia as a subjective sense of gaps in one's memory for autobiographical information or experiences, or for blocks of time that have passed, where such lapses cannot be attributed to ordinary forgetfulness.)*
1. Have you ever felt as if there were gaps in your memory? IF YES: Can you describe that experience? (Can you describe an example of the type of gaps you experienced? What made you aware of the gaps?)	**Gaps in Memory** O Unclear O No O Yes O Inconsistent *(Amnesia may be described as "blank periods," "blackouts," or "spacing out.")* Description:
2. How often are you aware of gaps in your memory? (How often have you experienced gaps in your memory?) (Rate the most frequent period.)	**Frequency of Memory Gaps** O unable to state frequency O rarely (up to 4 isolated episodes) O occasionally (up to 4 episodes per year) O frequently (5 or more episodes per year) O monthly (up to 3 episodes per month) O daily/weekly (4 or more episodes per month) O persistent gaps in memory
2a. Have you ever felt as if your memories were vague or unclear? (Have you ever had other problems with your memory?) IF YES: Can you describe that experience? (What type of memory problems have you had? What made you aware of these problems?) How often does that occur?	**Other Memory Problems** O Unclear O No O Yes O Inconsistent Description:

Cite as: Steinberg M: The SCID-D Interview: Dissociation Assessment in Therapy, Forensics, and Research. Washington, DC, American Psychiatric Association Publishing, 2023

2b. Have other people ever told you that you had gaps or problems with your memory? IF YES: What have other people told you?	**Told by Others About Memory Problems** ○ Unclear　○ No　○ Yes　○ Inconsistent Description:
2c. How often have you been told that you had gaps or problems with your memory? (Rate the most frequent period.)	**Frequency of Told Memory Problems** ○ unable to state frequency ○ rarely (up to 4 isolated episodes) ○ occasionally (up to 4 episodes per year) ○ frequently (5 or more episodes per year) ○ monthly (up to 3 episodes per month) ○ daily/weekly (4 or more episodes per month)
3. Have there ever been hours or days that seemed to be missing or that you couldn't account for? (Have you ever been unable to remember specific events or time periods in your life?) IF YES: How much time was missing? (What made you aware of the missing time?) *or* What events or time periods were you unable to recall? (What is that experience like?)	**Lost Time or Amnesia for Specific Events** ○ Unclear　○ No　○ Yes　○ Inconsistent Description:
4. How often have you experienced missing time? (How often have you lost hours or days?) (Rate the most frequent period.)	**Frequency of Lost Time** ○ unable to state frequency ○ rarely (up to 4 isolated episodes) ○ occasionally (up to 4 episodes per year) ○ frequently (5 or more episodes per year) ○ monthly (up to 3 episodes per month) ○ daily/weekly (4 or more episodes per month)
5. What is the longest period of time you've ever lost? (What is the longest period of time that was missing?)	**Longest Period of Lost Time** ○ unclear ○ minutes ○ hours ○ days ○ weeks ○ months ○ years

6. Has there ever been a time in which you had difficulty remembering your daily activities? IF YES: Can you describe what that was like? (How often does that occur?)	**Difficulty Remembering Daily Activities** ○ Unclear ○ No ○ Yes ○ Inconsistent Description:
7. **Have you ever found yourself in a place and been unable to remember how or why you went there?** IF YES: Can you describe what occurred and where you found yourself?	**Unable to Remember Going to a Place** ○ Unclear ○ No ○ Yes ○ Inconsistent Description:
8. How often does that occur? (Rate the most frequent period.)	**Frequency of Amnesia for Going to a Place** ○ unable to state frequency ○ rarely (up to 4 isolated episodes) ○ occasionally (up to 4 episodes per year) ○ frequently (5 or more episodes per year) ○ monthly (up to 3 episodes per month) ○ daily/weekly (4 or more episodes per month)
9. **Have you ever traveled away from your home or work unexpectedly and been unable to remember information about yourself or your past?** IF YES: Can you describe what occurred? (Where did you find yourself? What information were you unable to remember? How often has that occurred?)	**Dissociative Amnesia With Fugue** ○ Unclear ○ No ○ Yes ○ Inconsistent Description:
10. Were you aware of a reason for your travel?	**Reason for Travel** ○ Unclear ○ No ○ Yes ○ Inconsistent

11. Have you ever found yourself in a place away from your home or work and been unable to remember who you were? IF YES: Can you describe what occurred and where you found yourself?	**Loss of Identity With Travel** ○ Unclear ○ No ○ Yes ○ Inconsistent Description:
12. How often does that occur? (Rate the most frequent period.)	**Frequency of Identity Loss With Travel** ○ unable to state frequency ○ rarely (up to 4 isolated episodes) ○ occasionally (up to 4 episodes per year) ○ frequently (5 or more episodes per year) ○ monthly (up to 3 episodes per month) ○ daily/weekly (4 or more episodes per month)
13. During the time when you traveled to _____, did you (place of travel described in #9 or #11) experience any confusion or changes in your usual identity? IF YES: Can you describe the confusion (or changes in your identity)?	**Identity Confusion or Changes During Travel** ○ unclear ○ did not experience changes in identity ○ experienced confusion regarding identity ○ experienced loss of identity ○ experienced alteration in identity Description:
14. How often does that occur? (Rate the most frequent period.)	**Frequency Identity Confusion During Travel** ○ unable to state frequency ○ rarely (up to 4 isolated episodes) ○ occasionally (up to 4 episodes per year) ○ frequently (5 or more episodes per year) ○ monthly (up to 3 episodes per month) ○ daily/weekly (4 or more episodes per month)
15. Have you ever been unable to remember your name, age, address, or other important personal information? IF YES: What information did you forget?	**Amnesia for Personal Information** ○ Unclear ○ No ○ Yes ○ Inconsistent Description:

16. How often does that occur? (Rate the most frequent period.)	**Frequency of Amnesia for Personal Information** ○ unable to state frequency ○ rarely (up to 4 isolated episodes) ○ occasionally (up to 4 episodes per year) ○ frequently (5 or more episodes per year) ○ monthly (up to 3 episodes per month) ○ daily/weekly (4 or more episodes per month)
*17.	*Dissociative Amnesia criteria are rated after completing the entire interview.*
If the client's elaborations provide evidence of clinically meaningful amnesia, continue with question 18. Otherwise, skip ahead to question 38 (Depersonalization section, page 29).	
18. How old were you the first time you experienced ——————— ? (endorsed symptoms of amnesia)	**Age at First Symptom** ○ unclear ○ early childhood (up to age 6) ○ childhood (ages 7–12) ○ adolescence (ages 13–19) ○ young adult (ages 20–30) ○ adult (over age 31)
19. When was the last time you experienced ——————— ? (endorsed symptoms of amnesia)	**Age at Last Noted Symptom** ○ unclear ○ early childhood (up to age 6) ○ childhood (ages 7–12) ○ adolescence (ages 13–19) ○ young adult (ages 20–30) ○ adult (over age 31)
20. (Rate the most recent episode)	**Most Recent Amnesia Episode** ○ unclear ○ prior to past year ○ past year ○ past month

21. When you experience _____, **does that** (endorsed symptoms of amnesia or fugue)' **ever interfere with your social relationships, work, or ability to function?** IF YES: How does it interfere (with your relationships, work, or ability to function)?	**Amnesia Interferes With Functioning** ○ Unclear ○ No ○ Yes ○ Inconsistent Description:
*22. When you experience _____, is it related to (endorsed symptoms of amnesia or fugue)' (or triggered by) stressful experiences? IF YES: Can you describe a stressful experience that seemed related to _____? (symptoms of amnesia/fugue)	**Associated With Stress** ○ unclear ○ not associated with stress ○ sometimes associated with stress ○ usually associated with stress Description:
23. When you experience _____, **does that** (endorsed symptoms of amnesia or fugue)' **cause you discomfort (or distress)?**	**Causes Discomfort or Distress** ○ unclear ○ does not cause distress ○ sometimes causes distress ○ usually causes distress
*23a. When you have memories of past events, does that ever cause you discomfort (or distress)? (Do the memories ever interfere with your relationships or ability to function?) IF YES: What is that experience like? (How do the memories interfere?)	**Memories Interfere With Functioning or Cause Discomfort or Distress** ○ unclear ○ no ○ prefers not to think about past memories ○ yes
If client does not have a history of substance use, medical illness, or head trauma, skip ahead to question 38 (Depersonalization section, page 29). *If client has a history of amnesia and substance use, medical illness, or head trauma, continue with question 24 (Rule Out Organic Etiology).*	

AMNESIA
Rule Out Organic Etiology

If there is no history of substance use, medication effect, head trauma, or other organic etiology, skip this section and continue with question 38 (Depersonalization section, page 29).	
24. Just before you experienced _____, **were you using or withdrawing from drugs?** (endorsed amnesia symptoms) IF YES: Can you describe what occurred? What drugs had you been using?	**Drugs of Abuse** ○ Unclear ○ No ○ Yes ○ Inconsistent Description:
25. Just before you experienced _____, **were you drinking?** (endorsed amnesia symptoms) IF YES: Can you describe what occurred? What were you drinking, and how much?	**Drinking** ○ Unclear ○ No ○ Yes ○ Inconsistent Description:
26. Did you have any head trauma that could have caused _____? (endorsed amnesia symptoms) IF YES: Can you describe what occurred? (How often has that occurred?) During that time, did you see a doctor? IF YES: What did the doctor say was the cause of your _____? (endorsed amnesia symptoms)	**Head Trauma** ○ Unclear ○ No ○ Yes ○ Inconsistent Description:

27. Did you have a medical condition or were you using medication that could have caused _____? _(endorsed amnesia symptoms) IF YES: What medical illness did you have? (What medication do you believe caused your symptoms?) During that time, did you see a doctor? IF YES: What did the doctor say was the cause of your _____? _(endorsed amnesia symptoms)	**Medical Illness or Medication Adverse Effect** ○ Unclear ○ No ○ Yes ○ Inconsistent *(Dissociative amnesia is excluded if the client's amnesia occurs exclusively during or after a seizure, i.e., postictal amnesia.)* Description:
27a. Just before you experienced _____, **were you suffering** _(endorsed amnesia symptoms) **from lack of sleep/exhaustion?** IF YES: What led to your lack of sleep? (How much sleep did you get? How long were you sleep deprived? Did you see a doctor? IF YES: What did the doctor say was the cause of your _____?) _(endorsed amnesia symptoms)	**Sleep Deprivation/Exhaustion** ○ Unclear ○ No ○ Yes ○ Inconsistent Description:
If YES to any of the questions 24–27, continue with question 28. IF NO to questions 24–27, skip to question 38 (Depersonalization section, page 29).	
28. Have you ever experienced _____ **when you were not** _(endorsed symptoms of amnesia) **using (or experiencing)** _____? _(endorsed substance, illness, exhaustion, head trauma) IF YES: **29.** How often has that occurred? (Rate the most frequent period.)	**Amnesia (Without Organic Etiology)** ○ Unclear ○ No ○ Yes ○ Inconsistent **Amnesia Frequency (Without Organic Etiology)** ○ unclear ○ rarely (up to 4 isolated episodes) ○ occasionally (up to 4 episodes per year) ○ frequently (5 or more episodes per year) ○ monthly (up to 3 episodes per month) ○ daily/weekly (4 or more episodes per month)

*30.	(Dissociative Amnesia criteria are rated after completing the entire interview.)
Rule Out Organic Etiology: Dissociative Fugue *If the client endorsed fugue episodes, continue with question 31.* *If the client denied fugue episodes, skip to question 38 (Depersonalization section, page 29).*	
31. Just before you experienced **_____ were you using or** (endorsed fugue symptoms) **withdrawing from any drugs?** IF YES: Can you describe what occurred? What drugs had you been using?	**Drug Use Before Fugue** O Unclear O No O Yes O Inconsistent Description:
32. Just before you experienced **_____ were you drinking?** (endorsed fugue symptoms) IF YES: Can you describe what occurred? What were you drinking, and how much?	**Drinking Before Fugue** O Unclear O No O Yes O Inconsistent Description:
33. Did you have any head trauma that could **have caused _____ ?** (endorsed fugue symptoms) IF YES: Can you describe what occurred? (How often has that occurred?) During that time, did you see a doctor? IF YES: What did the doctor say was the cause of your _____ ? (endorsed fugue symptoms)	**Head Trauma Associated With Fugue** O Unclear O No O Yes O Inconsistent Description:

34. Did you have a medical condition or were you using medication that could have caused _____? (endorsed fugue symptoms) IF YES: What medical illness did you have? (What medication do you believe caused your symptoms?) During that time, did you see a doctor? IF YES: What did the doctor say was the cause of your _____? (endorsed fugue symptoms)	**Medical Illness/Medication Caused Fugue** O Unclear O No O Yes O Inconsistent Description:
IF YES to any of the questions 31–34, continue with question 35. *IF NO to questions 31–34, skip to question 38 (Depersonalization section, page 29).*	

35. Have you ever experienced
 	
 _____ **when you were not**
 (endorsed fugue symptoms)
 using/suffering from
 	
 _____?
 (endorsed substance,illness,exhaustion,head trauma)
 	
     IF YES:
 	
 36. How often has that occurred?
 	
        (Rate the most frequent period.)
	Fugue (Without Organic Etiology)
	 O Unclear O No O Yes O Inconsistent
	
	 Frequency of Fugue (Without Organic Etiology)
	 O unclear
	 O rarely (up to 4 isolated episodes)
	 O occasionally (up to 4 episodes per year)
	 O frequently (5 or more episodes per year)
	 O monthly (up to 3 episodes per month)
	 O daily/weekly (4 or more episodes per month)

*37.	*Dissociative Fugue criteria are rated after completing the entire interview.*

DEPERSONALIZATION:
PAST AND CURRENT SYMPTOMS

Some people have experiences that feel very real to them but are difficult to explain to others. Now, I am going to ask you about some of those experiences.	*(For clinical assessment of dissociation, the author has defined depersonalization as a feeling of disconnection from oneself (e.g., from one's feelings, thoughts, behavior, or body), or a sense of being an outside observer of one's self.)*
38. Have you ever felt that you were watching yourself from a point outside (or inside) of your body, as if you were seeing yourself from a distance (or watching a movie of yourself)? IF YES: Can you describe that experience?	**Watching Yourself From a Distance** ○ Unclear ○ No ○ Yes ○ Inconsistent Description:
39. How often have you had that experience? (Rate the most frequent period.)	**Frequency of Watching Self From a Distance** ○ unclear ○ rarely (up to 4 isolated episodes) ○ occasionally (up to 4 episodes per year) ○ frequently (5 or more episodes per year) ○ monthly (up to 3 episodes per month) ○ daily/weekly (4 or more episodes per month)
40. Have you ever had the feeling that you were a stranger to yourself? IF YES: What is that experience like? (How often does that occur?)	**Stranger to Yourself** ○ Unclear ○ No ○ Yes ○ Inconsistent Description:
40a. Have you ever had difficulty recognizing yourself when looking in a mirror? IF YES: Can you describe that experience? How often does that occur?	**Difficulty Recognizing Self in Mirror** ○ Unclear ○ No ○ Yes ○ Inconsistent Difficulty recognizing one's self in the mirror may indicate underlying depersonalization.* Description:

* Steinberg M, Schnall M: *The Stranger in the Mirror: Dissociation—The Hidden Epidemic*. New York, HarperCollins, 2001.

Cite as: Steinberg M: The SCID-D Interview: Dissociation Assessment in Therapy, Forensics, and Research. Washington, DC, American Psychiatric Association Publishing, 2023

40b. Have you ever felt as if you were losing your sense of self? (Have you ever felt that you didn't have an identity?)
 	
   IF YES: What is that experience like?
   How often have you had that experience?
	Losing Sense of Self
	○ Unclear ○ No ○ Yes ○ Inconsistent
	
	Description:

41. Have you ever felt as if a part of your body or your whole being was foreign to you? IF YES: What is that experience like? (How often does that occur?)	**Part of Body Was Foreign** ○ Unclear ○ No ○ Yes ○ Inconsistent Description:
42. Have you ever felt as if part of your body was disconnected (detached) from the rest of your body? (Have you ever felt as if part of your body or whole body was numb or that you couldn't feel pain?) IF YES: What is that experience like? (How often does that occur?)	**Part of Body Was Disconnected or Numb** ○ Unclear ○ No ○ Yes ○ Inconsistent Description:
43. Have you ever felt as if part of your body or your whole body disappeared? (Have you ever felt as if you were fading away or invisible?) IF YES: What is that experience like? (How often does that occur?)	**Part of Body Disappeared** ○ Unclear ○ No ○ Yes ○ Inconsistent Description:

44. Have you ever felt as if part of your body or your whole being was unreal?

    IF YES: What is that experience like?

Body Felt Unreal

○ Unclear   ○ No   ○ Yes   ○ Inconsistent

Description:

---

45. How often have you had that experience?

    (Rate the most frequent period.)

Frequency of Feeling Body Felt Unreal

○ unclear

○ rarely (up to 4 isolated episodes)

○ occasionally (up to 4 episodes per year)

○ frequently (5 or more episodes per year)

○ monthly (up to 3 episodes per month)

○ daily/weekly (4 or more episodes per month)

---

46. Have you ever felt as if you were going through the motions of living but the real you was far away from what was happening to you? (Have you ever felt disconnected [detached] from your feelings or behavior?)

    IF YES: What is that experience like?
    (How often does that occur?)

Disconnected From Real Self or Feelings

○ Unclear   ○ No   ○ Yes   ○ Inconsistent

Description:

---

47. Have you ever felt as if you were two different people, one going through the motions of life and the other observing?

    IF YES: What is that experience like?

Part Observing

○ Unclear   ○ No   ○ Yes   ○ Inconsistent

Description:

---

48. How often have you had that experience?

    (Rate the most frequent period.)

Frequency of Part Observing

○ unclear

○ rarely (up to 4 isolated episodes)

○ occasionally (up to 4 episodes per year)

○ frequently (5 or more episodes per year)

○ monthly (up to 3 episodes per month)

○ daily/weekly (4 or more episodes per month)

*49. Have you ever felt as if your arms or legs were bigger or smaller than usual or were changing size? IF YES: What is that experience like?	**Arms or Legs Changed Size** ○ Unclear ○ No ○ Yes ○ Inconsistent Description:
*50. Have you ever heard yourself talking and felt that you were not the one choosing the words? (Have you ever felt as if words seem to flow from your mouth as if they were not in your control?) IF YES: What is that experience like? (How often does that occur?)	**Not Choosing One's Words** ○ Unclear ○ No ○ Yes ○ Inconsistent Description:
*51. Have you ever felt as if your behavior was not in your control? IF YES: What is that experience like? Can you share an example of when you felt your behavior was not in your control? (How often does that occur?)	**Behavior Was Not in One's Control** ○ Unclear ○ No ○ Yes ○ Inconsistent Description:
*52. Have you ever felt as if your emotions were not in your control? IF YES: What is that experience like? (How often does that occur?)	**Emotions Not in One's Control** ○ Unclear ○ No ○ Yes ○ Inconsistent Description:
*53. Have you ever felt as if you were a puppet under someone else's control? IF YES: What is that experience like?	**Like a Puppet** ○ Unclear ○ No ○ Yes ○ Inconsistent Description:

*54. (Rate most severe frequency)	**Frequency of Most Severe Depersonalization** ○ unclear ○ rarely (up to 4 isolated episodes) ○ occasionally (up to 4 episodes per year) ○ frequently (5 or more episodes per year) ○ monthly (up to 3 episodes per month) ○ daily/weekly (4 or more episodes per month)
If the client's elaborations provide evidence of clinically meaningful depersonalization, continue with question 55. Otherwise, skip ahead to question 79 (Derealization section, page 39).	
*55. What is the longest period of time ——————————————— ever lasted? _(endorsed symptoms of depersonalization)	**Longest Episode of Depersonalization** ○ unclear ○ minutes ○ hours (one or more) ○ days (one or more) ○ weeks (one or more) ○ months (one or more) ○ years (one or more)
*56. Does each experience of ——————————————— last for about _(endorsed symptoms of depersonalization) the same amount of time or does it vary in duration?	**Duration of Depersonalization Episodes** ○ unclear ○ variable duration ○ similar in duration
*57. Does each experience of ——————————————— begin suddenly _(endorsed symptoms of depersonalization) or gradually?	**Onset of Depersonalization** ○ unclear ○ usually sudden ○ variable onset ○ usually gradual
*58–59.	*Depersonalization diagnostic criteria are rated after completing the entire interview.*

60. How old were you when you first experienced————————————**?** (endorsed symptoms of depersonalization)	**Age at Onset of Depersonalization** ○ unclear ○ early childhood (up to age 6) ○ childhood (ages 7–12) ○ adolescence (ages 13–19) ○ young adult (ages 20–30) ○ adult (over age 31)
61. How old were you the last time that you experienced ————————————**?** (endorsed symptoms of depersonalization)	**Age at Last Depersonalization** ○ unclear ○ early childhood (up to age 6) ○ childhood (ages 7–12) ○ adolescence (ages 13–19) ○ young adult (ages 20–30) ○ adult (over age 31)
62.	**Most Recent Depersonalization Episode** ○ unclear ○ prior to past year ○ past year ○ past month
63. When you experience ————————————, **does that** (endorsed symptoms of depersonalization) **ever interfere with your social relationships, work, or ability to function?** IF YES: How does it interfere (with your relationships, work, or ability to function)?	**Depersonalization Interferes With Functioning** ○ Unclear ○ No ○ Yes ○ Inconsistent Description:
*64. When you experience ———————————— **is it related to** (endorsed symptoms of depersonalization) **(or triggered by) stress?**	**Associated With Stress** ○ unclear ○ not associated with stress ○ sometimes associated with stress ○ usually associated with stress

65. When you experience _____, **does that** (endorsed symptoms of depersonalization), **cause you discomfort (or distress)?**	**Causes Discomfort or Distress** ○ unclear ○ does not cause distress ○ sometimes causes distress ○ usually causes distress
*66.	*Depersonalization diagnostic criteria are rated after completing the entire interview.*
If the client's elaborations provide evidence of clinically meaningful depersonalization, continue with question 67. Otherwise, skip ahead to question 79 (Derealization section, page 39).	
67. When you experienced _____, **were you having any** (endorsed depersonalization), **other psychological problems?** IF YES: What type of problems did you have? (Did you see a doctor for those problems? IF YES: What did your doctor say?)	**Other Symptoms** ○ Unclear　　○ No　　○ Yes　　○ Inconsistent Description:
68. Do you have frequent panic attacks? IF YES: What are your panic attacks like? How often do you have panic attacks?	**Frequent Panic Attacks** ○ Unclear　　○ No　　○ Yes　　○ Inconsistent Description:
IF YES to panic attacks, continue with question 69. *IF NO panic attacks and no history of substance use, medical illness, or head trauma, skip to question 79 (Derealization section, page 39).* *IF NO panic attacks and there is a history of substance use, medical illness, or head trauma, skip to question 72 (Rule Out Organic Etiology, page 37).*	

69. Are the _____ related to your
(panic attack symptoms)

experiences of _____?
(endorsed depersonalization)

Related Symptoms

○ Unclear ○ No ○ Yes ○ Inconsistent

IF YES:

70. In what way are they related? How often are
they related?

Are the Symptoms Related?

○ unclear

○ not related

○ sometimes related

○ usually related

*If symptoms are related, continue with question 71.
If symptoms are not related, skip to question 72
(Rule Out Organic Etiology, page 37).*

71. Do you usually feel _____ first
(panic attack symptoms)

and then feel _____ or is it the
(endorsed depersonalization)

reverse?

Which Symptom Occurs First?

○ unclear

○ usually feels panic attacks first

○ sometimes feels panic first

○ usually experiences depersonalization first

71a. Have you ever experienced

_____ when you were not
(endorsed depersonalization)

experiencing panic attacks?

IF YES: How often does that occur?

Depersonalization (Without Panic)

○ Unclear ○ No ○ Yes ○ Inconsistent

Description:

*If client does not have a history of substance use,
medical illness, or head trauma, skip ahead to
question 79 (Derealization section, page 39).*

*If client has a history of depersonalization <u>and</u> a
history of substance use, medical illness, or head
trauma, continue with question 72 (Rule Out
Organic Etiology).*

DEPERSONALIZATION

Rule Out Organic Etiology

If there is no history of substance use, medication effect, head trauma, or organic etiology, skip this section and continue with question 79 (Derealization section, page 39).	
72. Just before you experienced _____, **were you** (endorsed depersonalization symptoms) **using or withdrawing from drugs?** IF YES: Can you describe what occurred? What drugs had you been using?	**Drugs of Abuse** ○ Unclear ○ No ○ Yes ○ Inconsistent Description:
73. Just before you experienced _____, **were you** (endorsed depersonalization symptoms) **drinking?** IF YES: Can you describe what occurred? What were you drinking, and how much?	**Drinking** ○ Unclear ○ No ○ Yes ○ Inconsistent Description:
74. Did you have any head trauma that could have caused _____? (endorsed depersonalization symptoms) IF YES: Can you describe what occurred? (How often has that occurred?) During that time, did you see a doctor? IF YES: What did the doctor say was the cause of your _____? (endorsed depersonalization symptoms)	**Head Trauma** ○ Unclear ○ No ○ Yes ○ Inconsistent Description:
75. Did you have a medical condition or were you using medication that could have caused _____? (endorsed depersonalization symptoms) IF YES: What medical illness did you have? (What medication do you believe caused your symptoms?) During that time, did you see a doctor? IF YES: What did the doctor say was the cause of _____? (endorsed depersonalization)	**Medical Illness or Medication Adverse Effect** ○ Unclear ○ No ○ Yes ○ Inconsistent Description:

75a. Just before you experienced _____, **were you** (endorsed depersonalization symptoms) **suffering from lack of sleep/exhaustion?** IF YES: What led to your lack of sleep? (How much sleep did you get? How long were you sleep deprived? Did you see a doctor? IF YES: What did the doctor say was the cause of your _____?) (endorsed depersonalization symptoms)	**Sleep Deprivation/Exhaustion** ○ Unclear ○ No ○ Yes ○ Inconsistent Description:
75b. Did you experience _____ **immediately before** (endorsed depersonalization) **falling asleep or waking up?** IF YES: Can you describe that experience?	**Hypnagogic or Hypnopompic State** ○ Unclear ○ No ○ Yes ○ Inconsistent Description:
If YES to any of the questions 72–75b, continue with question 76. *If NO to questions 72–75b, skip to question 79 (Derealization section, page 39).*	
76. Have you ever experienced _____ **when you were** (endorsed depersonalization symptoms) **not using (or experiencing)** _____? (endorsed substance, illness, exhaustion, head trauma) IF YES: **77. How often has that occurred?** (Rate the most frequent period.)	**Depersonalization (Without Organic Etiology)** ○ Unclear ○ No ○ Yes ○ Inconsistent **Frequency of Depersonalization (Without Organic Etiology)** ○ unclear ○ rarely (up to 4 isolated episodes) ○ occasionally (up to 4 episodes per year) ○ frequently (5 or more episodes per year) ○ monthly (up to 3 episodes per month) ○ daily/weekly (4 or more episodes per month)
*78.	*(Depersonalization diagnostic criteria are rated after completing the entire interview.)*

DEREALIZATION:
PAST AND CURRENT SYMPTOMS

Now I'll be asking you questions about how your surroundings and other people feel to you.	*(For clinical assessment of dissociation, the author has defined derealization as a feeling of disconnection from one's surroundings [e.g., people or surroundings feel as if they are unfamiliar, unreal, or distorted].)*
79. Have you ever felt as if familiar surroundings or people you knew seemed unfamiliar or unreal? IF YES: What is that experience like? (Can you describe who or what seemed unfamiliar or unreal?)	**Experienced Derealization** ○ Unclear ○ No ○ Yes ○ Inconsistent Description:
80. How often have you had that experience? (Rate the most frequent period.)	**Frequency of Derealization** ○ unclear ○ rarely (up to 4 isolated episodes) ○ occasionally (up to 4 episodes per year) ○ frequently (5 or more episodes per year) ○ monthly (up to 3 episodes per month) ○ daily/weekly (4 or more episodes per month)
81. Have you ever felt as if your surroundings or other people were fading away or dream-like? (Have your surroundings or other people ever appeared distorted, or changed in size?) IF YES: What is that experience like? (How often does that occur? How long does it last?)	**Perceptual Distortions** ○ Unclear ○ No ○ Yes ○ Inconsistent *(Varied perceptual distortions including visual disturbances have been described in association with derealization, including visual snow and tunnel vision.)* Description:

81a. Have you ever felt as if you were disconnected (or detached) from other people or your surroundings? IF YES: What is that experience like?	**Disconnected From People or Surroundings** ○ Unclear ○ No ○ Yes ○ Inconsistent Description:
81b. How often have you felt disconnected (or detached) from other people or your surroundings? (Rate the most frequent period.)	**Frequency of Detachment From Surroundings** ○ unclear ○ rarely (up to 4 isolated episodes) ○ occasionally (up to 4 episodes per year) ○ frequently (5 or more episodes per year) ○ monthly (up to 3 episodes per month) ○ daily/weekly (4 or more episodes per month)
82. Have you ever been unable to recognize close friends, relatives, or your own home? IF YES: What is that experience like? (How often does that occur?)	Unable to Recognize Friends, Relatives, **Home** ○ Unclear ○ No ○ Yes ○ Inconsistent Description:
83. Have you ever felt as if close friends, relatives, or your own home seemed strange or foreign? IF YES: What is that experience like? (How often does that occur?)	**People or Surroundings Were Foreign** ○ Unclear ○ No ○ Yes ○ Inconsistent Description:
84. Have you ever felt puzzled as to what is real and what is unreal in your surroundings? IF YES: What is that experience like?	**Puzzled About What Is Real/Unreal** ○ Unclear ○ No ○ Yes ○ Inconsistent Description:

85. How often does that occur? (Rate the most frequent period.)	**Rate Frequency of Most Severe Derealization** ○ unclear ○ rarely (up to 4 isolated episodes) ○ occasionally (up to 4 episodes per year) ○ frequently (5 episodes or more per year) ○ monthly (up to 3 episodes per month) ○ daily/weekly (4 or more episodes per month)
If client's elaborations provide evidence of clinically meaningful derealization, continue with question 86. Otherwise, skip ahead to question 101 (Identity Confusion section, page 45).	
*86. What is the longest period of time that ——————————————— ever lasted? _(endorsed symptoms of derealization)	**Longest Episode of Derealization** ○ unclear ○ minutes ○ hours (one or more) ○ days (one or more) ○ weeks (one or more) ○ months (one or more) ○ years (one or more)
*87. Does each experience of ——————————————— last for about _(endorsed symptoms of depersonalization) the same amount of time each time or does it vary in duration?	**Duration of Derealization Episodes** ○ unclear ○ variable duration ○ similar in duration
88. How old were you when you first **experienced** ———————————————? _(endorsed symptoms of derealization)	**Age at First Symptom** ○ unclear ○ early childhood (up to age 6) ○ childhood (ages 7–12) ○ adolescence (ages 13–19) ○ young adult (ages 20–30) ○ adult (over age 31)
89. How old were you the last time that you **experienced** ———————————————? _(endorsed symptoms of derealization)	**Age at Last Symptom** ○ unclear ○ early childhood (up to age 6) ○ childhood (ages 7–12) ○ adolescence (ages 13–19) ○ young adult (ages 20–30) ○ adult (over age 31)

*90. (Rate the most severe frequency)	**Rate Most Recent Derealization Episode** ○ unclear ○ prior to past year ○ past year ○ past month
91. When you experience **_____, does that ever** (endorsed symptoms of derealization), **interfere with your social relationships, work,** **or ability to function?** IF YES: How does it interfere (with your relationships, work, or ability to function?)	**Interferes with Functioning** ○ Unclear ○ No ○ Yes ○ Inconsistent Description:
*92. When you experience _____, is it related to (or (endorsed symptoms of derealization), triggered by) stress?	**Associated With Stress** ○ unclear ○ not associated with stress ○ sometimes associated with stress ○ usually associated with stress
93. When you experience **_____, does that cause** (endorsed symptoms of derealization), **you discomfort or distress?**	**Causes Discomfort or Distress** ○ unclear ○ does not cause distress ○ sometimes causes distress ○ usually causes distress
*94.	*(Derealization diagnostic criteria are rated after completing the entire interview.)*
If client does not have a history of substance use, medical illness, or head trauma, skip ahead to question 101 (Identity Confusion section, page 45). *If client has a history of derealization and a history of substance use, medical illness, or head trauma, continue with question 95 (Rule Out Organic Etiology).*	

DEREALIZATION
Rule Out Organic Etiology

If there is no history of substance use, medication effect, head trauma, or possible organic etiology, skip this section and continue with question 101 (Identity Confusion section, page 45).	
95. Just before you experienced _____**, were you using or withdrawing from drugs?** (endorsed derealization symptoms) IF YES: Can you describe what occurred? What drugs (or medications) had you been using?	**Drugs of Abuse** O Unclear O No O Yes O Inconsistent Description:
96. Just before you experienced _____**, were you drinking?** (endorsed derealization symptoms) IF YES: Can you describe what occurred? What were you drinking, and how much?	**Drinking** O Unclear O No O Yes O Inconsistent Description:
97. Did you have any head trauma that could have caused _____**?** (endorsed derealization symptoms) IF YES: Can you describe what occurred? (How often has that occurred?) During that time, did you see a doctor? IF YES: What did the doctor say was the cause of your _____? (endorsed derealization symptoms)	**Head Trauma** O Unclear O No O Yes O Inconsistent Description:

98. Did you have a medical condition or were you using medication that could have caused _____? _(endorsed derealization symptoms) IF YES: What medical illness did you have? (What medication caused your symptoms?) Did you see a doctor? IF YES: What did the doctor say caused your _____? _(endorsed symptoms)	**Medical Illness or Medication Adverse Effect** ○ Unclear ○ No ○ Yes ○ Inconsistent Description:
98a. Just before you experienced _____ **were you suffering** _(endorsed derealization symptoms) **from lack of sleep/exhaustion?** IF YES: What led to your lack of sleep? (How much sleep did you get? How long were you sleep deprived? Did you see a doctor? IF YES: What did the doctor say caused your _____?) _(endorsed symptoms)	**Sleep Deprivation/Exhaustion** ○ Unclear ○ No ○ Yes ○ Inconsistent Description:
98b. Did you experience _____ **immediately** _(endorsed derealization symptoms) **before falling asleep or waking up?** IF YES: Can you describe that experience?	**Hypnagogic or Hypnopompic State** ○ Unclear ○ No ○ Yes ○ Inconsistent Description:
If YES to any of the questions 95–98b, continue with question 99. If NO to questions 95–98b, skip to question 101 (Identity Confusion section, page 45).	
99. Have you ever experienced _____ **when you were not** _(endorsed derealization symptoms) **using/suffering from** _____? _(endorsed substance, illness, exhaustion, head trauma) IF YES: **100.** How often has that occurred? (Rate the most frequent period.)	**Derealization (Without Organic Etiology)** ○ Unclear ○ No ○ Yes ○ Inconsistent **Frequency of DR (Without Organic Etiology)** ○ unclear ○ rarely (up to 4 isolated episodes) ○ occasionally (up to 4 episodes per year) ○ frequently (5 or more episodes per year) ○ monthly (up to 3 episodes per month) ○ daily/weekly (4 or more episodes per month)

IDENTITY CONFUSION:
PAST AND CURRENT SYMPTOMS

Sometimes a person's sense of self can help us understand what their life is like. I will now ask you questions about what it feels like to be you.	*(For clinical assessment of dissociation, the author has defined identity confusion as subjective feelings of uncertainty, puzzlement, or conflict or struggle regarding one's own identity.)*
101. Have you ever felt as if there was a struggle going on inside of you? IF YES: Can you describe the struggle? (What is that experience like?) How often does that occur?	**Internal Struggle** ○ Unclear ○ No ○ Yes ○ Inconsistent Description:
102. Have you ever felt as if there was a struggle going on inside of you about who you really are? IF YES: Can you describe the struggle? (Can you describe the different sides of the struggle?)	**Identity Struggle** ○ Unclear ○ No ○ Yes ○ Inconsistent Description:
103. How often does that occur? (Rate the most frequent period.)	**Frequency of Identity Struggle** ○ unclear ○ rarely (up to 4 isolated episodes) ○ occasionally (up to 4 episodes per year) ○ frequently (5 or more episodes per year) ○ monthly (up to 3 episodes per month) ○ weekly or daily (4 or more episodes per month)
104. Is the struggle accompanied by any physical symptoms? IF YES: What physical symptoms do you experience?	**Physical Symptoms With Identity Struggle** ○ Unclear ○ No ○ Yes ○ Inconsistent *(Varied somatic symptoms, including headaches, visual changes, muscle tension, tics, other involuntary movements, or pain, often co-occur with identity struggles.)* Description:

Cite as: Steinberg M: The SCID-D Interview: Dissociation Assessment in Therapy, Forensics, and Research. Washington, DC, American Psychiatric Association Publishing, 2023

105. Have you ever felt confused or uncertain as to who you are? (Have you ever felt that you didn't know who you were?) IF YES: What is that experience like?	**Confusion/Lack of Identity** ○ Unclear ○ No ○ Yes ○ Inconsistent Description:
IF YES to questions 102 or 105, continue with 105a. IF NO, continue with question 105b.	
105a. Adolescents and other people may have periods of confusion or struggles about their identity. How does your confusion (or struggles) compare with that experienced by others you know? (How is it similar, and how does it differ?)	**Similar to Identity Confusion in Adolescents?** ○ unclear ○ confusion is similar ○ confusion is different Description:

105b. Have you ever felt as if there were different parts or sides of you?
 	
    IF YES: What is that experience like?
    Can you describe the different parts or sides?
	Different Parts of Identity
	○ Unclear ○ No ○ Yes ○ Inconsistent
	
	Description:

105c. How often have you felt as if there were different parts (or sides) of you? (Rate the most frequent period.)	**Frequency of Different Parts of Identity** ○ unclear ○ rarely (up to 4 isolated episodes) ○ occasionally (up to 4 episodes per year) ○ frequently (5 or more episodes per year) ○ monthly (up to 3 episodes per month) ○ weekly or daily (4 or more episodes per month)

105d. Have you ever felt as if there was a childlike part or side of you? 　IF YES: What is that experience like? Can you describe what seems childlike about that part (or side)?	**Childlike Part or Side** ○ Unclear　　○ No　　○ Yes　　○ Inconsistent Description:
105e. How often do you feel as if there is/was a childlike part or side of you? 　　(Rate the most frequent period.)	**Frequency of Childlike Part or Side** ○ unclear ○ rarely (up to 4 isolated episodes) ○ occasionally (up to 4 episodes per year) ○ frequently (5 or more episodes per year) ○ monthly (up to 3 episodes per month) ○ weekly or daily (4 or more episodes per month)
If the client's elaborations provide evidence of clinically meaningful identity confusion, continue with question 106. Otherwise, skip ahead to question 113 (Identity Alteration section, page 49).	
106. What is the longest period of time ——————————————————— **ever lasted?** _(endorsed symptoms of identity confusion)	**Longest Period of Identity Confusion** ○ unclear ○ minutes ○ hours (one or more) ○ days (one or more) ○ weeks (one or more) ○ months (one or more) ○ years (one or more)
107. How old were you when you first experienced ——————————————**?** _(endorsed symptoms of identity confusion)	**Age at Onset of Identity Confusion** ○ unclear ○ early childhood (up to age 6) ○ childhood (ages 7–12) ○ adolescence (ages 13–19) ○ young adult (ages 20–30) ○ adult (over age 31)

108. How old were you the last time that you experienced _____? _(endorsed symptoms of identity confusion)_	**Age at Last Identity Confusion** O unclear O early childhood (up to age 6) O childhood (ages 7–12) O adolescence (ages 13–19) O young adult (ages 20–30) O adult (over age 31)
*109.	**Rate Most Recent Identity Confusion Episode** O unclear O prior to past year O past year O past month
110. When you experience _____, **does that** _(endorsed symptoms of identity confusion)_ **ever interfere with your social relationships, work, or ability to function?** IF YES: How does it interfere (with your relationships, work, or ability to function)?	**Interferes With Functioning** O Unclear O No O Yes O Inconsistent Description:
*111. When you experience _____, **is it** _(endorsed symptoms of identity confusion)_ **related to (or triggered by) stress?**	**Associated With Stress** O unclear O not associated with stress O sometimes associated with stress O usually associated with stress
112. When you experience _____, **does that** _(endorsed symptoms of identity confusion)_ **cause you discomfort (or distress)?**	**Causes Discomfort or Distress** O unclear O does not cause distress O sometimes causes distress O usually causes distress

IDENTITY ALTERATION:
PAST AND CURRENT SYMPTOMS

Sometimes a person's behaviors and experiences can help us understand more about their life. I'll now ask you questions about some of your experiences.	*(For clinical assessment of dissociation, the author defines identity alteration as observable behavior associated with shifts or alterations in one's identity or personality states.)*
113. Have you ever felt as if, or found yourself behaving as if, you were still a child? (Have you ever been told you were behaving like a child?) IF YES: What is that experience like? Can you share an example of how you felt like or behaved like a child? How often does that occur?	**Childlike Feelings or Behavior** O Unclear O No O Yes O Inconsistent Description:
113a. Have you ever found yourself acting out of character or not like your usual self? IF YES: What is that experience like? Can you describe how you acted differently? How often does that occur?	**Acted Out of Character** O Unclear O No O Yes O Inconsistent Description:
114. Have you ever felt as if, or acted as if, you were a different person? IF YES: What is that experience like? (Can you describe how you felt/acted differently?)	**Felt or Acted Differently** O Unclear O No O Yes O Inconsistent Description:
115. How often have you had that experience? (Rate the most frequent period.)	**Frequency of Acting Differently** O unclear O rarely (up to 4 isolated episodes) O occasionally (up to 4 episodes per year) O frequently (5 or more episodes per year) O monthly (up to 3 episodes per month) O daily/weekly (4 or more episodes per month)

116. Have you ever been told by others that you seem like a different person?

IF YES: Who said that and what did they mean? (When did that occur? How often does that occur?)

Told That You Seem Different
○ Unclear   ○ No   ○ Yes   ○ Inconsistent

Description:

---

117. How often have you been told that you seem like a different person?

(Rate the most frequent period.)

Frequency of Being Told You Seem Different
○ unclear
○ rarely (up to 4 isolated episodes)
○ occasionally (up to 4 episodes per year)
○ frequently (5 or more episodes per year)
○ monthly (up to 3 episodes per month)
○ daily/weekly (4 or more episodes per month)

---

118. Have you ever referred to yourself (or been told by others that you referred to yourself) by different names (other than name changes due to marriage)?

IF YES: Can you describe what that experience is like? Can you share any of those names? (When were you first aware of using those names?)

Different Name (proper noun or symbolic)
○ Unclear   ○ No   ○ Yes   ○ Inconsistent

Description:

---

119. How often have you referred to yourself (or been told by others that you referred to yourself) by different names?

(Rate the most frequent period.)

Frequency of Using Different Names
○ unclear
○ rarely (up to 4 isolated episodes)
○ occasionally (up to 4 episodes per year)
○ frequently (5 episodes or more per year)
○ monthly episodes (up to 3 per month)
○ daily/weekly (4 or more episodes per month)

---

120. Have other people referred to you by different names (other than name changes due to marriage)?

IF YES: Can you share any of those names?

Others Refer to You by Different Names
○ Unclear   ○ No   ○ Yes   ○ Inconsistent

Description:

121. How often does that occur? (Rate the most frequent period.)	**Frequency of Others Using Different Names** ○ unclear ○ rarely (up to 4 isolated episodes) ○ occasionally (up to 4 episodes per year) ○ frequently (5 or more episodes per year) ○ monthly (up to 3 episodes per month) ○ daily/weekly (4 or more episodes per month
122. Have you ever found things in your possession that seemed to belong to you, but you could not remember how you acquired them? IF YES: What did you find in your possession?	**Amnesia for Possessions** ○ Unclear ○ No ○ Yes ○ Inconsistent Description:
123. How often does that occur? (Rate the most frequent period.)	**Frequency of Amnesia for Possessions** ○ unclear ○ rarely (up to 4 isolated episodes) ○ occasionally (up to 4 episodes per year) ○ frequently (5 or more episodes per year) ○ monthly (up to 3 episodes per month) ○ daily/weekly (4 or more episodes per month)
124. Have you ever felt as if you were possessed? IF YES: Can you describe what that experience is like? Who did you feel possessed by? (How often have you felt possessed?)	**Felt Possessed** ○ Unclear ○ No ○ Yes ○ Inconsistent (Common possession states include feeling as if one's behavior or speech is controlled by another person, spirit, supernatural being or force.) Description:
124a. Have you ever felt as if you were in a trance? (Have you ever experienced a change in your awareness of your surroundings [or state of consciousness] that was not in your control?) IF YES: Can you describe what that experience is like? (How often has that occurred? How long did you feel as if you were in a trance?)	**Trance State/Altered Consciousness** ○ Unclear ○ No ○ Yes ○ Inconsistent Description:

125. What is the longest period of time _____ ever lasted? (endorsed symptoms of identity alteration)	**Longest Period of Symptoms** ○ unclear ○ minutes ○ hours ○ days ○ weeks ○ months ○ years
126. How old were you when you first experienced _____? (endorsed symptoms of identity alteration)	**Age at Onset of Identity Alteration** ○ unclear ○ early childhood (up to age 6) ○ childhood (ages 7–12) ○ adolescence (ages 13–19) ○ young adult (ages 20–30) ○ adult (over age 31)
127. How old were you the last time that you experienced _____? (endorsed symptoms of identity alteration)	**Age at Last Identity Alteration** ○ unclear ○ early childhood (up to age 6) ○ childhood (ages 7–12) ○ adolescence (ages 13–19) ○ young adult (ages 20–30) ○ adult (over age 31)
*128. (Rate the most severe frequency.)	**Rate Most Recent Identity Alteration Episode** ○ unclear ○ prior to past year ○ past year ○ past month

129. When you experience	Interferes With Functioning
_____, does that ever (endorsed symptoms of identity alteration) **interfere with your social relationships, work, or ability to function?** IF YES: How does it interfere (with your relationships, work, or ability to function)?	○ Unclear ○ No ○ Yes ○ Inconsistent Description:
***130.** When you experience _____, is it related to (endorsed symptoms of identity alteration) (or triggered by) stress?	**Associated With Stress** ○ unclear ○ not associated with stress ○ sometimes associated with stress ○ usually associated with stress
131. When you experience **_____, does that cause** (endorsed symptoms of identity alteration) **you discomfort (or distress)?**	**Causes Discomfort or Distress** ○ unclear ○ does not cause distress ○ sometimes causes distress ○ usually causes distress
If client's elaborations provide evidence of clinically meaningful identity confusion or alteration, continue with question 132 (Rule Out Organic Etiology). Otherwise, skip ahead to question 134 (Associated Features of Identity Confusion and Identity Alteration section, page 59).	

IDENTITY ALTERATION
Rule Out Organic Etiology

If there is no history of substance use, medication effect, head trauma, or organic etiology, skip this section and continue with question 134 on page 59 (Associated Features of Identity Confusion and Identity Alteration).	
132. Just before you experienced ─────────────────────── **were you using** (endorsed identity alteration symptoms) **or withdrawing from drugs, alcohol, or a medication?** IF YES: Can you describe what occurred? What drugs/alcohol had you been using? (What medication do you believe caused your symptoms?)	**Drugs, Alcohol, or Medication Effect** ○ Unclear ○ No ○ Yes ○ Inconsistent Description:
132a. Did you have a medical condition or head trauma that could have caused ───────────────────────? (endorsed identity alteration symptoms) IF YES: What medical illness or trauma did you have? Did you see a doctor? IF YES: What did the doctor say was the cause of ───────────────────────? (endorsed identity alteration symptoms)	**Medical Illness or Medication Adverse Effect** ○ Unclear ○ No ○ Yes ○ Inconsistent Description:

132b. Just before you _____ **were you** (endorsed identity alteration symptoms) **suffering from lack of sleep/exhaustion?** IF YES: What led to your lack of sleep? (How much sleep did you get? How long were you sleep deprived? Did you see a doctor? IF YES: What did the doctor say was the cause of your _____?) (endorsed identity alteration symptoms)	**Sleep Deprivation/Exhaustion** ○ Unclear　　○ No　　○ Yes　　○ Inconsistent Description:
If YES to any of the questions 132–132b, continue with question 133. *If NO to questions 132–132b, skip to question 134 (Associated Features of Identity Confusion and Identity Alteration, page 59).*	
133. Have you ever experienced _____ **when you were** (endorsed identity alteration symptoms) **not using/experiencing** _____? (endorsed substance, illness, exhaustion, head trauma) IF YES: **133a.** How often has that occurred? 　　　(Rate the most frequent period.)	**Identity Alteration (Without Organic Etiology)** ○ Unclear　　○ No　　○ Yes　　○ Inconsistent **Frequency of Identity Alteration (Without Organic Etiology)** ○ unclear ○ rarely (up to 4 isolated episodes) ○ occasionally (up to 4 episodes per year) ○ frequently (5 or more episodes per year) ○ monthly (up to 3 episodes per month) ○ daily/weekly (4 or more episodes per month)

PART III:
FURTHER EXPLORATION OF
IDENTITY CONFUSION & ALTERATION

ASSOCIATED FEATURES OF
IDENTITY CONFUSION AND IDENTITY ALTERATION
MOOD CHANGES; FLASHBACKS; INTERNAL DIALOGUES, VOICES, AND INTRUSIVE THOUGHTS

134. Have you ever experienced frequent or rapid mood changes? (Has anyone ever told you that your mood changes frequently or rapidly?) IF YES: What is that experience like? (What type of mood changes do you experience?) How often does that occur?	**Frequent or Rapid Mood Changes** ○ Unclear ○ No ○ Yes ○ Inconsistent Description:
134a. Have you experienced mood changes that seem out of proportion to the situation? IF YES: What is that experience like? Can you share an example of when you felt as if your mood was out of proportion to the situation? How often does that occur?	**Mood Changes That Seem Excessive** ○ Unclear ○ No ○ Yes ○ Inconsistent Description:
135. Have you ever experienced (or been told of) changes in your capabilities or ability to function? IF YES: What is that experience like? How often does that occur?	**Changes in Ability to Function** ○ Unclear ○ No ○ Yes ○ Inconsistent Description:

Cite as: Steinberg M: The SCID-D Interview: Dissociation Assessment in Therapy, Forensics, and Research. Washington, DC, American Psychiatric Association Publishing, 2023

136. Have you ever felt as if you were re-experiencing (reliving) past memories or feelings as if they were occurring in the present? (Have you ever felt as if you were living in the past?) IF YES: What is that experience like? (Would you feel comfortable sharing an example of when you felt like you were reliving past feelings or memories?)	**Flashbacks/Re-experiencing the Past** ○ Unclear ○ No ○ Yes ○ Inconsistent Description:
137. How often does that occur? (Rate the most frequent period.)	**Frequency of Re-experiencing the Past** ○ unclear ○ rarely (up to 4 isolated episodes) ○ occasionally (up to 4 episodes per year) ○ frequently (5 or more episodes per year) ○ monthly (up to 3 episodes per month) ○ daily/weekly (4 or more episodes per month)
138. Have you ever talked to yourself or had inner dialogues with yourself? IF YES: Can you describe what you experienced? (Can you share an example of what was said?) How often do you talk to yourself or have dialogues? (Is the content of the self-talk or dialogues usually supportive, critical, or a mixture of both?)	**Talked to Self or Inner Dialogues** ○ Unclear ○ No ○ Yes ○ Inconsistent Description:
138a. Have you ever experienced an inner voice or unwanted thoughts that were critical of you or other people? IF YES: Can you share an example of what you experienced? How often does that occur?	**Critical Voice/Intrusive Thoughts** ○ Unclear ○ No ○ Yes ○ Inconsistent Description:

138b. Have you ever experienced an inner voice or unwanted thoughts that seem childlike? IF YES: Can you share an example of what you experienced? How often does that occur?	**Childlike Voice/Intrusive Thoughts** ○ Unclear ○ No ○ Yes ○ Inconsistent Description:
IF YES to dialogues, or childlike or critical voices (138–138b), continue with question 139. *IF NO to dialogues, or childlike or critical voices (138–138b), skip to page 65 (Follow-Up Sections).*	
139. Do you experience the **_____ silently?** (dialogues, unwanted thoughts, or voice)	**Dialogues, Intrusive Thoughts, or Voices Silently** ○ Unclear ○ No ○ Yes ○ Inconsistent
140. Do you ever talk to yourself out loud? (Do you hear the _____ (dialogues, unwanted thoughts, or voice) as if it's spoken out loud?)	**Dialogues, Intrusive Thoughts, or Voices Aloud** ○ Unclear ○ No ○ Yes ○ Inconsistent
*141. Do you ever have written dialogues with yourself? IF YES: Can you describe an example of a written dialogue?	**Written Dialogues** ○ Unclear ○ No ○ Yes ○ Inconsistent
*142. Does your handwriting ever change noticeably? IF YES: What changes are you aware of?	**Change in Handwriting** ○ Unclear ○ No ○ Yes ○ Inconsistent Description:

143. How often do you experience

_____ ?
(dialogues, unwanted thoughts, or voices)

(Rate the most frequent period.)

Frequency: Self-talk, Intrusive Thoughts, Voices
- ○ unclear
- ○ rarely (up to 4 isolated episodes)
- ○ occasionally (up to 4 episodes per year)
- ○ frequently (5 or more episodes per year)
- ○ monthly (up to 3 episodes per month)
- ○ daily/weekly (4 or more episodes per month)

Questions 144 through 158 are optional since they are not necessary for diagnostic purposes. Skip ahead to page 65 (Follow-up Sections) unless there is a particular interest to further explore voices, dialogues, or intrusive thoughts.

*144. Are the _____
(dialogues, unwanted thoughts, or voice)
similar to hearing voices? (Can you hear both sides of the conversation/dialogue? Does it feel as if there is an auditory component to the conversation/dialogues?)

Similar to Voices
○ Unclear   ○ No   ○ Yes   ○ Inconsistent

*145. Are the _____ similar to
(describe dialogues/voice)
thoughts?

Similar to Thoughts
○ Unclear   ○ No   ○ Yes   ○ Inconsistent

*146. Does it feel as if they occur inside your head (or outside)?

Dialogues/Voices Inside or Outside Head
- ○ unclear
- ○ usually outside
- ○ both inside and outside
- ○ usually inside

*147. Are the _____ related to (or
(describe dialogues/voice)
triggered by) stress?

Associated With Stress
- ○ unclear
- ○ not associated with stress
- ○ sometimes associated with stress
- ○ usually associated with stress

*148. When you experience ―――――――― (describe dialogues/voice) does this cause you discomfort (or distress)?	**Causes Discomfort or Distress** ○ unclear ○ does not cause distress ○ sometimes causes distress ○ usually causes distress
*149. Have you ever experienced having several conversations, dialogues, or voices occurring at the same time (silently or out loud)? IF YES: What is that like?	**Has Several Dialogues/Voices** ○ Unclear ○ No ○ Yes ○ Inconsistent Description:
IF YES to several conversations or voices occurring at the same time (question 149), continue with question 150. *IF NO, skip ahead to page 65 (Follow-Up Sections).*	
*150. Are the conversations/dialogues similar to hearing voices?	**Several Dialogues Similar to Voices** ○ Unclear ○ No ○ Yes ○ Inconsistent
*151. Are the ―――――――― (describe several dialogues/voices) similar to thoughts?	**Several Dialogues Similar to Thoughts** ○ Unclear ○ No ○ Yes ○ Inconsistent
*152. Does it feel as if they occur inside your head (as opposed to outside)?	**Several Voices Inside or Outside Head** ○ unclear ○ usually outside ○ both inside and outside ○ usually inside
*153. Do you experience the ―――――――― silently? (describe several dialogues/voices)	**Several Dialogues/Voices Are Silent** ○ Unclear ○ No ○ Yes ○ Inconsistent
*154. Do you experience the ―――――――― out loud? (describe several dialogues/voices)	**Several Dialogues/Voices Are Out Loud** ○ Unclear ○ No ○ Yes ○ Inconsistent

*155. Do you ever have written dialogues?	**Several Written Dialogues/Voices** ○ Unclear ○ No ○ Yes ○ Inconsistent
*156. How often do you have several (simultaneous) dialogues or voices? (Rate the most frequent period.)	**Frequency of Several Dialogues/Voices** ○ unclear ○ rarely (up to 4 isolated episodes) ○ occasionally (up to 4 episodes per year) ○ frequently (5 or more episodes per year) ○ monthly (up to 3 episodes per month) ○ daily/weekly (4 or more episodes per month)
*157. Are the _____ related (describe several dialogues/voices) to (or triggered by) stress?	**Several Dialogues Associated With Stress** ○ unclear ○ not associated with stress ○ sometimes associated with stress ○ usually associated with stress
*158. When you experience _____, does that cause you (describe several dialogues/voices), discomfort (or distress)?	**Several Dialogues Cause Discomfort or Distress** ○ unclear ○ does not cause distress ○ sometimes causes distress ○ usually causes distress

FOLLOW-UP SECTIONS:
IDENTITY CONFUSION AND ALTERATION

The nature and extent of an individual's identity struggles, and conflicting aspects of self are evaluated further in the Follow-Up sections listed in Table 1 below. Additional information elicited by administering the follow-up sections allows the interviewer to better assess the constellation of symptoms supporting the presence or absence of a more complex dissociative disorder (e.g., Dissociative Identity Disorder, or Other Specified Dissociative Disorder under DSM-5-TR, or Partial Dissociative Disorder under ICD-11).

The first nine symptom areas listed in Table 1 are relevant to both DSM or ICD classification, and refer to symptoms that may have been endorsed by the client during the first part of the SCID-D administration. If the client endorsed and described clinically significant symptoms listed in Table 1, then continue the interview by asking the corresponding Follow-Up questions listed in the table for that symptom area. Otherwise, if the client has *not* endorsed any of the symptom areas, you may end the interview here. It is recommended that the interviewer begin with the Follow-Up section of the symptom area that seems most clinically significant based upon the client's presentation so far. The interviewer should personalize the questions in each Follow-Up section by incorporating descriptive information that the client had described previously. For diagnostic purposes, it is usually unnecessary to administer more than two Follow-Up sections. For use in therapy, administering as many Follow-Up sections the client's endorsed symptoms call for can provide additional therapeutically meaningful information.

The last Follow-Up section was designed specifically to facilitate distinguishing DID from Partial DID for ICD-11 diagnosis, and can be pursued *after* completing one or more other follow-up sections in Table 1.

Table 1: Endorsed Symptoms and Their Corresponding Follow-Up Section

Follow-Up Sections for Endorsed Symptoms	Initial Symptom Questions	Follow-Up Questions	Page
Parts of Self and Identity Confusion	101–112, Entire interview	159–169	67
Mood Changes	134	170–180	73
Depersonalization	38–77	181–191	77
Different Names	118–121	192–201	81
Voices, Dialogues, and Intrusive Thoughts	138–158	202–211	87
Childlike Part	105d–e, 113, 138b	212–222	91
Flashbacks	136–137	223–233	95
Different Person	114–117	234–244	101
Possession or Trance	124, 124a	245–258	105
ICD-11 Specific: Distinguishing DID from Partial DID	Entire interview	258.01–258.12	111

PARTS OF SELF AND IDENTITY CONFUSION FOLLOW-UP

In this section, the interviewer can explore manifestations of identity confusion or of parts of self, including the emotional, cognitive, behavioral, addictive, or somatic alterations or shifts associated with parts of self. Questions should be personalized to refer to the parts of self or the identity confusion that the client described. Examples of parts of self that can be explored include, but are not limited to, emotional (e.g., sad, angry or terrified parts); cognitive/behavioral (e.g., critical, obsessive-compulsive parts, or self-harming parts); addictive (e.g., eating disordered, binging, purging, alcohol/drug using, or sexually addictive parts); and/or somatic (e.g., pseudoseizures, or other alterations in sensory-motor functioning). Examples of personalized fill-in phrases include a part of you that "is terrified," a part of you that "eats food and then purges," a part of you that "cuts your arm," a part of you that "uses alcohol," a part of you that "has seizure-like movements in your arms and legs." This section can be repeated for each part of self that the interviewer is exploring.

Earlier you mentioned that you've experienced a part of you that _____? Can you say anything more about that part? (describe part of self) (Earlier you mentioned that you've felt as if there is a struggle going on inside of you as to who you really are. Can you say anything more about the sides or parts of the struggle?)	Description:
159. Does it feel as if the part of you that _____ ever influences or controls the way you act, speak, feel, or think? (describe part of self) IF YES: In what way does _____ influence or control you? (describe part of self) (Does the way you _____ remind you of anyone you know, or of any past experience you have had? (act, speak, feel, or think) IF YES: Who does it remind you of? *or* What experience does it remind you of?)	**Influences Actions, Speech, Feelings, Thoughts** ○ Unclear ○ No ○ Yes ○ Inconsistent Description:

Cite as: Steinberg M: The SCID-D Interview: Dissociation Assessment in Therapy, Forensics, and Research. Washington, DC, American Psychiatric Association Publishing, 2023

160. Do you have a visual image that is associated with _____?
(describe part of self)
(Do you associate a facial expression, tone of voice, feeling, or movement with

_____?)
(describe part of self)

   IF YES: What is the

_____ like?
(image, expression, voice, feeling, etc.)

   (Does the _____
(image, expression, voice, feeling, etc.)
remind you of anyone you know, or of any past experience you have had?

   IF YES: Who does it remind you of? *or*
What experience does it remind you of?)

| **Image, Voice, etc., Associated With Part** |
| O Unclear O No O Yes O Inconsistent |
| Description: |

---

161. Is there an age (or age range) that you associate with _____?
(describe part of self)

   IF YES: What age or age range?
(What is the youngest age that you associate

with _____?)
(describe part of self)

| **Age(s) Associated With Part** |
| O Unclear O No O Yes O Inconsistent |
| Description: |

---

162. Is there a name (actual or symbolic) that you associate with _____?
(describe part of self)

   IF YES:

   163. What name(s) are you aware of?

Name Associated With Part
O Unclear O No O Yes O Inconsistent

Aware of Names
O unclear
O has 1 or more nicknames or descriptive names
O has 1 other proper name (not nickname)
O has 2–5 other proper names
O has 6 or more proper names

164. Have you ever talked with or had inner dialogues with ―――――― (silently or out loud)? (describe part of self)	**Inner Talk or Dialogues** ○ Unclear ○ No ○ Yes ○ Inconsistent Description:
164a. Have you ever experienced unwanted thoughts or heard voices that you associate with ―――――― ? (describe part of self) IF YES to 164 or 164a: Can you share an example of what was said? (How often do you experience ――――――?) (inner talk, unwanted thoughts, or voices)	**Intrusive Thoughts or Voices** ○ Unclear ○ No ○ Yes ○ Inconsistent Description:
165. If ―――――― could speak, what (describe part of self) **might ―――――― say?** (describe part of self) (What might ―――――― say to help us (describe part of self) understand more about ――――――?) (describe part of self, or "you", or "your life")	Description:
If the client's responses suggest an identity disturbance, continue with question 165a. Otherwise, if there are no additional Follow-Up sections you wish to pursue (see page 65), you may end the interview here.	
165a. What does ―――――― need to feel (describe part of self) **more at peace?** (What do you need to feel more at peace with ――――――?) (describe part of self) *and/or* (What does ――――――― need to ("your adult self" or "your compassionate self") feel more at peace with ――――――?) (describe part of self)	Description:

*166. Does it feel as if ——————— could
 (describe part of self)
 talk with a therapist directly?
 	
    IF YES: What might ——————— say?
    (describe part of self)
	Talk With Therapist
	 O Unclear O No O Yes O Inconsistent
	 Description:

167. Does it feel as if ——————— has
 (describe part of self)
 different memories, behaviors, feelings, or
 beliefs than your own, or does it feel similar?
 (Or, does it sometimes feel similar and sometimes
 different?)
 	
    IF DIFFERENT: In what way are they
    different?
	Different Memories, Behaviors, Feelings, etc.
	 O unclear
	 O feels similar
	 O sometimes feels different
	 O feels different
	
	 Description:

168. Does it feel as if ——————— is
 (describe part of self)
 a part of your personality, or does it feel
 separate? (Or, does it sometimes feel separate,
 and sometimes a part of your personality?)
 	
    IF YES (to feels separate): Can you describe
    what you mean when you say it feels separate?
	Separate or Part of Personality
	 O unclear
	 O part of personality
	 O sometimes feels separate, sometimes not
	 O feels separate
	
	 Description:

169.	**Summary: Personality States**
	 O Inadequate information
	 O Lacks evidence of 2 or more personality states
	 O Suspect 2 or more personality states, but
	    distinctness is unclear
	 O Appears to have 2 or more distinct personality
	    states (i.e., with related alterations in affect,
	    memory, behavior, cognition, and/or sensory-
	    motor control)

169a.	**Summary: Shifts in Executive Control/Agency**
	○ Inadequate information
	○ Lacks evidence of shifts in executive control
	○ Shifts in control seem less-than-marked
	○ Marked shifts in executive control
If the presence, absence, or type of dissociative disorder is clear, you may end the interview here. Otherwise, consider administering an additional Follow-Up section (see page 65).	

MOOD CHANGES FOLLOW-UP

Questions in this follow-up section should be personalized to refer to a mood that the client described. Examples of personalized fill-in phrases include your feelings of "rage," your feelings of "hopelessness," your feelings of being "overwhelmed," your feelings of "shame," your feelings of being "confused," "manic," or "guarded," etc. This section can be repeated for each mood that the interviewer is exploring.

Earlier you mentioned that you have experienced mood changes. Can you say anything more about the moods you experience?	Description:
170. Does it feel as if ―――― ever (describe mood) **influences or controls the way you act, speak, feel, or think?** IF YES: In what way does ―――― (describe mood) influence or control you? (Does the way you ―――― remind (act, speak, feel or think) you of anyone you know or of any past experience you have had? IF YES: Who does it remind you of? <u>or</u> What experience does it remind you of?)	**Influences Actions, Speech, Feelings, Thoughts** ○ Unclear ○ No ○ Yes ○ Inconsistent Description:
171. Do you have a visual image that is associated with ―――― ? (describe mood) (Do you associate a facial expression, tone of voice, sensation, or movement with ――――?) (describe mood) IF YES: What is the ―――― like? (image, expression, voice, sensation, etc.) (Does the ―――― (image, expression, voice, sensation, etc.) remind you of anyone you know, or of any past experience you have had? IF YES: Who does it remind you of? *or* What experience does it remind you of?)	**Image, Voice, etc., Associated With Mood** ○ Unclear ○ No ○ Yes ○ Inconsistent Description:

172. Is there an age (or age range) that you associate with $\underline{\hspace{2cm}}$ **?** (describe mood) IF YES: What age or age range? (What is the youngest age that you associate with $\underline{\hspace{2cm}}$?) (describe mood)	**Age(s) Associated With Mood** ○ Unclear ○ No ○ Yes ○ Inconsistent Description:
173. Is there a name (actual or symbolic) that you associate with $\underline{\hspace{2cm}}$ **?** (describe mood) IF YES: **174.** What names are you aware of?	**Name Associated With Moods** ○ Unclear ○ No ○ Yes ○ Inconsistent **Aware of Names** ○ unclear ○ has 1 or more nicknames or descriptive names ○ has 1 other proper name (not nickname) ○ has 2–5 other proper names ○ has 6 or more proper names
175. Have you ever talked with or had inner dialogues with $\underline{\hspace{2cm}}$ **(silently or out loud)?** (describe mood)	**Talked With or Dialogues** ○ Unclear ○ No ○ Yes ○ Inconsistent
175a. Have you ever experienced unwanted thoughts or heard voices that you associate with $\underline{\hspace{2cm}}$ **?** (describe mood) IF YES to 175 or 175a: Can you share an example of what was said? (Is the content of the $\underline{\hspace{3cm}}$ usually (inner talk, unwanted thoughts, or voices) supportive, critical, or a mixture of both?) (How often do you experience $\underline{\hspace{3cm}}$ with (inner talk, unwanted thoughts, or voices) $\underline{\hspace{2cm}}$?) (describe mood)	**Intrusive Thoughts or Voices** ○ Unclear ○ No ○ Yes ○ Inconsistent Description:

176. If ――――――― **could speak, what might** (describe mood) ――――――― **say?** (describe mood) (What might ――――――― say to help us (describe mood) understand more about ――――――――――――?) (describe mood, or "you" or "your life")	Description:
If the client's responses suggest an identity disturbance, continue with question 176a. Otherwise, if there are no additional Follow-Up sections you wish to pursue (see page 65), you may end the interview here.	
176a. What does ――――――― **need to feel** (describe mood) **more at peace?** (What do you need to feel more at peace with ―――――――?) (describe mood) *and/or* (What does ――――――――――――――― need to ("your adult self"/or "your compassionate self") feel more at peace with ―――――――?) (describe mood)	Description:
***177.** Does it feel as if ――――――― could talk (describe mood) with a therapist directly? IF YES: What might ――――――― say? (describe mood)	**Talk With Therapist** ○ Unclear ○ No ○ Yes ○ Inconsistent Description:

178. Does it feel as if _____ **has different** (describe mood) **memories, behaviors, feelings, or beliefs than** **your own, or does it feel similar?** (Or, does it sometimes feel similar and sometimes different?) IF YES: In what way are they different?	**Different Memories, Behaviors, or Feelings** ○ unclear ○ feels similar ○ sometimes feels different ○ feels different Description:

179. Does it feel as if _____ **is a part of**
 (describe mood)
 your personality, or does it feel separate? (Or
 does it sometimes feel separate, and sometimes a
 part of your personality?)
 	
    IF YES (to feels separate): Can you describe
    what you mean when you say it feels separate?
	Separate or Part of Personality
	 ○ unclear
	 ○ part of personality
	 ○ sometimes feels separate, sometimes not
	 ○ feels separate
	
	 Description:

180.	**Summary: Personality States**
	 ○ Inadequate information
	 ○ Lacks evidence of 2 or more personality states
	 ○ Suspect 2 or more personality states, but
	    distinctness is unclear
	 ○ Appears to have 2 or more distinct personality
	    states (i.e., with related alterations in affect,
	    memory, behavior, cognition, and/or sensory-
	    motor control)

180a.	**Summary: Shifts in Executive Control/Agency** ○ Inadequate information ○ Lacks evidence of shifts in executive control ○ Shifts in control seem less-than-marked ○ Marked shifts in executive control
If the presence, absence, or type of dissociative *disorder is clear, you may end the interview here.* *If more information is needed, continue with an* *additional Follow-Up section (see page 65).*	

DEPERSONALIZATION FOLLOW-UP

Questions in this follow-up section should be personalized to refer to the depersonalization experience that the client described. Examples of personalized fill-in phrases for DP experiences include feeling "emotionally numb," feeling "as if you are going through the motions of living," feeling "detached from your own feelings," and feeling "as if your hands are not your own," etc.

In addition to asking about a depersonalized experience, a "non-depersonalized" state of being (perhaps present before the onset of depersonalization) can be explored in this follow-up section. Examples of personalized fill-in phrases for the non-depersonalized experiences include feeling "the way you felt prior to feeling numb," feeling "in touch with your feelings," feeling "able to feel joy," etc.

Besides Depersonalization Disorder, depersonalization symptoms can indicate a more complex dissociative disorder, such as DID and OSDD, where depersonalization symptoms have been found to commonly co-occur with moderate to severe levels of the other four SCID-D symptoms.

Earlier you mentioned that you have had the experience of feeling _____ (describe DP experience). **Can you say anything more about that?** **Prior to experiencing** _____ (describe DP experience), **did you experience life differently?** IF YES: Can you describe what your life was like before you experienced _____ (describe DP experience). (Can you share an example of how your life was different?)	Description:
181. Do you have a visual image that is associated with feeling _____ (describe DP experience)? (Do you associate a facial expression, tone of voice, feeling, or movement with _____ (describe DP experience)?) IF YES: What is the _____ (image, voice, feeling, etc.) like? (Does the _____ (image, voice, feeling, etc.) remind you of anyone you know, or of any past experience you have had? IF YES: Who does it remind you of? *or* What experience does it remind you of?)	**Image, Voice, etc., of Depersonalized State** ○ Unclear ○ No ○ Yes ○ Inconsistent Description:

Cite as: Steinberg M: The SCID-D Interview: Dissociation Assessment in Therapy, Forensics, and Research. Washington, DC, American Psychiatric Association Publishing, 2023

182. Is there an age (or age range) that you associate with feeling _____? *(describe DP experience)* IF YES: What age or age range?	**Age(s) Associated With Depersonalized State** ○ Unclear ○ No ○ Yes ○ Inconsistent Description:
183. Is there a name (actual or symbolic) that you associate with feeling _____? *(describe DP experience)* IF YES: **184.** What name(s) are you aware of?	**Name(s) Associated With Depersonalized State** ○ Unclear ○ No ○ Yes ○ Inconsistent **Aware of Names** ○ unclear ○ has 1 or more nicknames or descriptive names ○ has 1 other proper name (not nickname) ○ has 2–5 other proper names ○ has 6 or more proper names
185. Does feeling _____ **ever** *(describe DP experience)* **influence or control the way you act, speak, feel, or think?** IF YES: In what way does _____ *(describe DP experience)* influence or control you? (When you feel _____, does that remind you of *(describe DP experience)* anyone you know or of any past experience you have had? IF YES: Who does it remind you of? *or* What experience does it remind you of?)	**Influences Actions, Speech, Feelings, Thoughts** ○ Unclear ○ No ○ Yes ○ Inconsistent Description:
186. Have you ever talked with or had inner dialogues (silently or out loud) associated with _____? *(describe DP experience)*	**Talked With or Dialogues** ○ Unclear ○ No ○ Yes ○ Inconsistent
186a. Have you ever experienced unwanted thoughts or heard voices that you associate **with** _____? *(describe DP experience)* IF YES to 186 or 186a: Can you share an example of what was said? (How often do you experience _____ *(inner talk, unwanted thoughts, or voices)* with _____?) *(describe DP experience)*	**Intrusive Thoughts or Voices** ○ Unclear ○ No ○ Yes ○ Inconsistent Description:

187. If the feelings associated with

_____ **could speak, what might**
(describe DP experience)
be said?

(What might the part of you that experiences

_____ say to help us understand
(describe DP experience)

more about _____?)
(describe DP state, or "you", or "your life")

Description:

If the client's responses are suggestive of an identity disturbance, continue with question 187a. Otherwise, if there are no additional Follow-Up sections you wish to pursue (see page 65), you may end the interview here.

187a. What does the part of you that

experiences _____ **need to feel**
(describe DP experience)
more at peace?

(What does

_____ need to
("your adult self" or "your compassionate self")

feel more at peace with _____?)
(describe DP experience)

Description:

---

*188. Does it feel as if the part of you that

experiences _____ could talk with
(describe DP experience)

a therapist directly?

   IF YES: Can you describe what might be said?

Talk With Therapist
○ Unclear   ○ No   ○ Yes   ○ Inconsistent

Description:

---

189. Does it feel as if the part of you that experiences _____ **has different** (describe DP experience) **memories, behaviors, feelings, or beliefs than your usual self (prior to DP), or does it feel similar?** (Or does it sometimes feel similar and sometimes different?) IF DIFFERENT: In what way are they different?	**Different Memories, Behaviors, Feelings, etc.** ○ unclear ○ not different ○ sometimes feels different ○ feels different Description:
190. Does it feel as if the part of you that experiences _____ **is a part of** (describe DP experience) **your personality, or does it feel separate?** (Or, does it sometimes feel separate and sometimes a part of your personality?) IF YES (to feels separate): Can you describe what you mean when you say it feels separate?	**Separate or Part of Personality** ○ unclear ○ part of personality ○ sometimes feels separate, sometimes not ○ feels separate Description:
191.	**Summary: Personality States** ○ Inadequate information ○ Lacks evidence of 2 or more personality states ○ Suspect 2 or more personality states, but distinctness is unclear ○ Appears to have 2 or more distinct personality states (i.e., with related alterations in affect, memory, behavior, cognition, and/or sensory-motor control)
191a.	**Summary: Shifts in Executive Control/Agency)** ○ Inadequate information ○ Lacks evidence of shifts in executive control ○ Shifts in control seem less-than-marked ○ Marked shifts in executive control
If the presence, absence, or type of dissociative disorder is clear, you may end the interview here. If more information is needed, continue with an additional Follow-Up section (see page 65).	

DIFFERENT NAMES FOLLOW-UP

Referring to oneself, or having others refer to one, by a nongiven name may indicate an identity disturbance, particularly when there is other evidence of identity confusion or alteration. Questions in this follow-up section should be personalized to refer to a name (either a proper noun or symbolic) that the client has used in referring to themself or that others have used in referring to the client (other than one's given name). Examples of personalized fill-in phrases for different names include "Sam," "Sally," "the monster," "the little," etc. This section can be repeated for each name that the interviewer is exploring.

192. Earlier you mentioned that you have referred to yourself (or other people referred to you) by ―――――――――. **Can you say** *(name provided by client)* **anything more about** ―――――――――**?** *(name provided by client)* (How do you understand why you referred to yourself [or been called by others] by this name?)	Description:
193. Does it feel as if ―――――――――― **ever** *(name provided by client)* **influences or controls the way you act, speak, feel, or think?** IF YES: In what way does ―――――――――― influence or control you? *(name provided by client)* (Does the way you ―――――――――― remind *(act, speak, feel, or think)* you of anyone you know or of any past experience you have had? IF YES: Who does it remind you of? *or* What experience does it remind you of?)	**Influences Actions, Speech, Feelings, Thoughts** ○ Unclear ○ No ○ Yes ○ Inconsistent Description:

Cite as: Steinberg M: The SCID-D Interview: Dissociation Assessment in Therapy, Forensics, and Research. Washington, DC, American Psychiatric Association Publishing, 2023

194. Do you picture —————————— **in a** (name provided by client) **particular way?** (Do you have a visual image that is associated with —————————— ?) (name provided by client) (Do you associate a facial expression, tone of voice, feeling, or movement with

—————————— ?) (name provided by client)

    IF YES: What is the

—————————— like? (image, expression, voice, feeling, etc.)

    (Does the —————————— (image, expression, voice, feeling, etc.) remind you of anyone you know, or of any past experience you have had?

    IF YES: Who does it remind you of? *or*

    What experience does it remind you of?)

Image, Voice, etc., Associated With Name
○ Unclear ○ No ○ Yes ○ Inconsistent

Description:

---

195. Do you think of a particular age (or age range) when you think of —————————— **?** (name provided by client) (Is there an age (or age range) that you associate with —————————— ?) (name provided by client)

    IF YES: What age or age range? (What is the youngest age that you associate with

—————————— ?) (name provided by client)

Age(s) Associated With Names
○ Unclear ○ No ○ Yes ○ Inconsistent

Description:

---

196. Have you ever talked with or had inner dialogues with —————————— **(silently or** (name provided by client) **out loud)?**

Inner Talk or Dialogues
○ Unclear ○ No ○ Yes ○ Inconsistent

196a. Have you ever experienced unwanted thoughts or heard voices that you associate with _____ **?**
(name provided by client)

    IF YES to 196 or 196a: Can you share an example of what was said?

    (How often do you experience

    _____
    (inner talk, dialogues, unwanted thoughts, or voices)

    with _____?)
        (name provided by client)

Intrusive Thoughts or Voices

○ Unclear   ○ No   ○ Yes   ○ Inconsistent

Description:

---

197. If _____ **could speak, what**
     (name provided by client)

might _____ **say?**
     (name provided by client)

(What might _____ say to help us
       (name provided by client)

understand more about

_____ ?)
(name provided by client, or "you" or "your life")

Description:

If the client's responses suggest an identity disturbance, continue with question 197a. Otherwise, if there are no additional Follow-Up sections you wish to pursue (see page 65), you may end the interview here.

197a. What does —————————— **need to**
(name provided by client)

feel more at peace?

(What do you need to feel more at peace with

—————————— ?)
(name provided by client)

and/or

(What does

——————————————— need to
("your adult self" or "your compassionate self")

feel more at peace with —————————— ?)
(name provided by client)

Description:

---

*198. Does it feel as if ——————————
(name provided by client)

could talk with a therapist directly?

    IF YES: What might —————————— say?
(name provided by client)

Talk With Therapist

O Unclear   O No   O Yes   O Inconsistent

Description:

---

199. Does it feel as if ——————————
(name provided by client)

has different memories, behaviors, feelings, or
beliefs than your own, or does it feel similar?
(Or, does it sometimes feel similar and sometimes
different?)

    IF YES: In what way are they different?

Different Memories, Behaviors, Feelings, etc.

O unclear

O feels similar

O sometimes feels different

O feels different

Description:

200. Does it feel as if _____ **is**
 (name provided by client)
 a part of your personality, or does it feel
 separate? (Or, does it sometimes feel separate,
 and sometimes a part of your personality?)
 	
    IF YES to feels separate: Can you describe
    what you mean when you say it feels separate?
	Separate or Part of Personality
	 ◯ unclear
	 ◯ part of personality
	 ◯ sometimes feels separate, sometimes not
	 ◯ feels separate
	 Description:

201.	**Summary: Personality States**
	 ◯ Inadequate information
	 ◯ Lacks evidence of 2 or more personality states
	 ◯ Suspect 2 or more personality states, but
	    distinctness is unclear
	 ◯ Appears to have 2 or more distinct personality
	    states (i.e., with related alterations in affect,
	    memory, behavior, cognition, and/or sensory-
	    motor control)

201a.	**Summary: Shifts in Executive Control/Agency** ◯ Inadequate information ◯ Lacks evidence of shifts in executive control ◯ Shifts in control seem less-than-marked ◯ Marked shifts in executive control
If the presence, absence, or type of dissociative *disorder is clear, you may end the interview here.* *If more information is needed, continue with an* *additional Follow-Up section (see page 65).*	

VOICES, DIALOGUES, AND INTRUSIVE THOUGHTS FOLLOW-UP

Questions in this follow-up section should be personalized to refer to a description of the voice, internal dialogues, or intrusive thoughts that the client had previously described. Examples of personalized fill-in phrases related to voices include "a voice that says you're a loser," "a voice that says you should hurt yourself," etc. Examples of personalized fill-in phrases related to intrusive thoughts include "thoughts that you should cut yourself," "thoughts that you should make sure you locked the door," "thoughts that you are unlovable," etc. This section can be repeated for each voice, dialogue, or intrusive thought that the interviewer is exploring.

Earlier you mentioned that you have experienced ⎯⎯⎯⎯⎯⎯⎯⎯⎯. (describe voice/intrusive thought) **Can you say anything more about that?** (How do you understand why you have experienced ⎯⎯⎯⎯⎯⎯⎯⎯⎯ ?) (describe voice/intrusive thought)	Description:
202. Does it feel as if ⎯⎯⎯⎯⎯⎯⎯⎯⎯ **ever influences or** (describe voice/intrusive thought) **controls the way you act, speak, feel, or think?** IF YES: In what way does it influence or control you? Does the way you ⎯⎯⎯⎯⎯⎯⎯ remind (act, speak, feel, or think) you of anyone you know or of any past experiences you have had? IF YES: Who does it remind you of? *or* What experience does it remind you of?)	**Influences Actions, Speech, Feelings, Thoughts** ○ Unclear ○ No ○ Yes ○ Inconsistent Description:

203. Do you have a visual image that you associate with ‾‾‾‾‾‾‾‾‾‾‾‾‾‾‾‾?
(describe voice/intrusive thought)
(Do you associate a facial expression, tone of voice, feeling, or movement with

‾‾‾‾‾‾‾‾‾‾‾‾‾‾‾‾‾‾?)
(describe voice/intrusive thought)

    IF YES: What is the

‾‾‾‾‾‾‾‾‾‾‾‾‾‾‾‾‾‾‾‾‾‾ like?
(image, expression, voice, feeling, etc.)

    (Does the ‾‾‾‾‾‾‾‾‾‾‾‾‾‾‾‾‾‾
(image, expression, voice, feeling, etc.)
remind you of anyone you know or of any past experience you have had?

    IF YES: Who does it remind you of? *or*
What experience does it remind you of?)

Image, etc., Associated With Voice/Intrusive Thoughts
○ Unclear ○ No ○ Yes ○ Inconsistent

Description:

---

204. Is there an age (or age range) that you associated with ‾‾‾‾‾‾‾‾‾‾‾‾‾‾‾‾?
(describe voice/intrusive thought)

    IF YES: What age or age range?
(What is the youngest age that you associate

with ‾‾‾‾‾‾‾‾‾‾‾‾‾‾‾‾ ?)
(describe voice/intrusive thought)

Age(s) Associated With Voice/Intrusive Thoughts
○ Unclear ○ No ○ Yes ○ Inconsistent

Description:

---

205. Do you have a name (actual or symbolic) that is associated with the

‾‾‾‾‾‾‾‾‾‾‾‾‾‾‾‾?
(describe voice/intrusive thought)

    IF YES:
206. What name(s) are you aware of?

Name(s) Associated With Voice/ Intrusive Thoughts
○ Unclear ○ No ○ Yes ○ Inconsistent

Aware of Names
○ unclear
○ has 1 or more nicknames or descriptive names
○ has 1 other proper name (not nickname)
○ has 2–5 other proper names
○ has 6 or more proper names

207. If _____ **could speak,** (describe voice/intrusive thought) **what might be said?**	Description:
(What might _____ say to (describe voice/intrusive thought) help us understand more about _____?) (describe dialogue/voice, or "you", or "your life")	
If the client's responses suggest an identity disturbance, continue with question 207a. Otherwise, if there are no additional Follow-Up sections you wish to pursue (see page 65), you may end the interview here.	
207a. What does _____ (describe voice/intrusive thought) **need to feel more at peace?** (What do you need to feel more at peace with _____ ?) (describe voice/intrusive thought) *and/or* (What does _____ need to ("your adult self" or "your compassionate self") feel more at peace with _____ ?) (describe voice/intrusive thought)	Description:
*208. Does it feel as if _____ could talk with a (describe voice/intrusive thought) therapist directly? IF YES: Can you describe what might be said?	**Talk With Therapist** ○ Unclear ○ No ○ Yes ○ Inconsistent Description:

209. Does it feel as if
 	
_____ **represents different**
(describe voice/intrusive thought)
memories, behaviors, feelings, or beliefs than
your own, or does it feel similar? (Or, does it
sometimes feel similar and sometimes different?)
 	
   IF DIFFERENT: In what way are they
   different?
	Different Memories, Behaviors, Feelings, etc.
	○ unclear
	○ feels similar
	○ sometimes feels different
	○ feels different
	
	Description:

210. Does it feel as if
 	
_____ **is a part of your**
(describe voice/intrusive thoughts)
personality, or does it feel separate?
(Or, does it sometimes feel separate and
sometimes a part of your personality?)
 	
   IF YES (to feels separate): Can you describe
   what you mean when you say it feels separate?
	Separate or Part of Personality
	○ unclear
	○ part of personality
	○ sometimes feels separate, sometimes not
	○ feels separate
	
	Description:

211.	**Summary: Personality States**
	○ Inadequate information
	○ Lacks evidence of 2 or more personality states
	○ Suspect 2 or more personality states, but
	   distinctness is unclear
	○ Appears to have 2 or more distinct personality
	   states (i.e., with related alterations in affect,
	   memory, behavior, cognition, and/or sensory-
	   motor control)

211a.	**Summary: Shifts in Executive Control/Agency** ○ Inadequate information ○ Lacks evidence of shifts in executive control ○ Shifts in control seem less-than-marked ○ Marked shifts in executive control
If the presence, absence, or type of dissociative *disorder is clear, you may end the interview here.* *If more information is needed, continue with an* *additional Follow-Up section (see page 65).*	

CHILDLIKE PART FOLLOW-UP

Questions in this follow-up section should be personalized to refer to the childlike part and/or its feelings, behaviors, or beliefs that the client described. Examples of personalized fill-in phrases include "the sad, helpless child," "the terrified child," "the innocent child that feels so alone," etc. This section can be repeated for each childlike part of self that the interviewer is exploring.

Earlier you mentioned that sometimes you feel as if (or behave as if) you were a child. Can you say anything more about that? (How do you understand why that occurs?)	Description:
212. Does it feel as if _____ (describe childlike part) **ever influences or controls the way you act, speak, feel, or think?** IF YES: In what way does it influence or control you? (Does the way you _____ (act, speak, feel, or think) remind you of anyone you know or of any past experiences you have had? IF YES: Who does it remind you of? *or* What experience does it remind you of?)	**Influences Actions, Speech, Feelings, Thoughts** ○ Unclear ○ No ○ Yes ○ Inconsistent Description:
213. Do you have a visual image that is associated with _____ (describe childlike part)**?** (Do you picture the child in a particular way?) (Are you aware of a facial expression, tone of voice, feeling, or sensation that you associate with _____ (describe childlike part)?) IF YES: What is the _____ (image, expression, voice, feeling, etc.) like?) (Does the _____ (image, expression, voice, feeling, etc.) remind you of anyone you know, or of any past experience you have had? IF YES: Who does it remind you of? *or* What experience does it remind you of?)	**Image, Voice, or Movement of Childlike Part** ○ Unclear ○ No ○ Yes ○ Inconsistent Description:

Cite as: Steinberg M: The SCID-D Interview: Dissociation Assessment in Therapy, Forensics, and Research. Washington, DC, American Psychiatric Association Publishing, 2023

214. Is there an age (or age range) that you associate with _____**?** (describe childlike part) IF YES: What age or age range? (What is the youngest age that you associate with _____**?)** (describe childlike part)	**Age(s) Associated With Childlike Part** ○ Unclear ○ No ○ Yes ○ Inconsistent Description:
215. Is there a name (actual or symbolic) that you associate with _____**?** (describe childlike part) IF YES: **216.** What names are you aware of?	**Name(s) Associated With Childlike Part** ○ Unclear ○ No ○ Yes ○ Inconsistent **Aware of Names** ○ unclear ○ has 1 or more nicknames or descriptive names ○ has 1 other proper name (not nickname) ○ has 2–5 other proper names ○ has 6 or more proper names
217. Have you ever talked with or had inner dialogues with _____ **(silently or** (describe childlike part) **out loud)?**	**Inner Talk** ○ Unclear ○ No ○ Yes ○ Inconsistent
217a. Have you ever experienced unwanted thoughts or heard voices that you associate with _____**?** (describe childlike part) IF YES to 217 or 217a: Can you share an example of what was said? (Is the content of the _____ usually (inner talk, unwanted thoughts, or voices) supportive, critical, or a mixture of both?) (How often do you experience _____ with (inner talk, unwanted thoughts, or voices) _____**?)** (describe childlike part)	**Intrusive Thoughts or Voices** ○ Unclear ○ No ○ Yes ○ Inconsistent Description:

218. If _____ **could speak, what**
　　(describe childlike part)

might _____ **say?**
　　　　(describe childlike part)

(What might _____ say to help us
　　　　　(describe childlike part)

understand more

_____?)
(describe childlike part, or "you", or "your life")

Description:

---

*If the client's responses suggest an identity
disturbance, continue with question 218a.
Otherwise, if there are no additional Follow-Up
sections you wish to pursue (see page 65), you
may end the interview here.*

218a. What does _____ **need to**
　　　　　　(describe childlike part)

feel more at peace?

(What do you need to feel more at peace with

_____?)
(describe childlike part)

and/or

(What does

_____ need to
("your adult self" or "your compassionate self")

feel more at peace with _____?)
　　　　　　　　　(describe childlike part)

Description:

---

*219. Does it feel as if _____
　　　　　　　　　　(describe childlike part)

could talk with a therapist directly?

　　IF YES: What might _____ say?
　　　　　　　　　　(describe childlike part)

Talk With Therapist

○ Unclear　　○ No　　○ Yes　　○ Inconsistent

Description:

---

220. Does it feel as if _____
(describe childlike part)
has different memories, behaviors, feelings, or beliefs than your own, or does it feel similar? (Or, does it sometimes feel similar and sometimes different?)

   IF DIFFERENT:
   In what way are they different?

Different Memories, Behaviors, Feelings, etc.
- O unclear
- O feels similar
- O sometimes feels different
- O feels different

Description:

---

221. Does it feel as if _____
(describe childlike part)
is a part of your personality, or does it feel separate? (Or, does it sometimes feel separate and sometimes a part of your personality?)

   IF YES to feels separate: Can you describe what you mean when you say it feels separate?

Separate or Part of Personality
- O unclear
- O part of personality
- O sometimes feels separate, sometimes not
- O feels separate

Description:

222.

Summary: Personality States
- O Inadequate information
- O Lacks evidence of 2 or more personality states
- O Suspect 2 or more personality states, but distinctness is unclear
- O Appears to have 2 or more distinct personality states (i.e., with related alterations in affect, memory, behavior, cognition, and/or sensory-motor control)

222a.

Summary: Shifts in Executive Control/Agency
- O Inadequate information
- O Lacks evidence of shifts in executive control
- O Shifts in control seem less-than-marked
- O Marked shifts in executive control

If the presence, absence, or type of dissociative disorder is clear, you may end the interview here. If more information is needed, continue with an additional Follow-Up section (see page 65).

FLASHBACK FOLLOW-UP

A flashback is the re-experiencing of past memories of an event as if they were occurring in the present. Flashbacks may also include re-experiencing the same emotions, behaviors, and sensations associated with the past event. Questions in this follow-up section should be personalized to refer to the description of the flashback state or event that the client described. Examples of possible personalized fill-in phrases include "being in combat," or "seeing the face of the person who raped you," or "memories of your cousin abusing you," etc.

Earlier you mentioned that you have felt as if you had re-experienced _____ **as** (describe flashback) **though it was occurring in the present. Can you say anything more about that?**	Description:
223. How old do you feel when you feel as if you're re-experiencing _____ **?** (describe flashback) (What age or age range?) (What is the youngest age that you associate with re-experiencing _____?) (describe flashback)	**Age(s) Associated With Flashback State** ○ Unclear ○ No ○ Yes ○ Inconsistent Description:
224. Do you have a visual image (of yourself or others) that is associated with re-experiencing _____ **?** (describe flashback) (Do you associate a facial expression, tone of voice, feeling, or movement with _____?) (describe flashback) IF YES: What is the _____ like? (image, expression, voice, feeling, etc.) (Does the _____ (image, expression, voice, feeling, etc.) remind you of anyone you know or of any past experience you have had? IF YES: Who does it remind you of? *or* What experience does it remind you of?)	**Image, Voice, etc., Associated With Flashback** ○ Unclear ○ No ○ Yes ○ Inconsistent Description:

225. Is there a name (actual or symbolic) that you associate with yourself when re-experiencing _(describe flashback)_**?**	**Name Associated With Flashback** ○ Unclear　　○ No　○ Yes　　○ Inconsistent Description:
IF YES: **226.** Are you able to share that name (or names)?	**Name(s) Used** ○ unclear ○ has 1 or more nicknames or descriptive names ○ has 1 other proper name (not nickname) ○ has 2–5 other proper names ○ has 6 or more proper names
227. Does it feel as if the part of you that re-experiences _(describe flashback)_ **ever influences or controls the way you act, speak, feel, or think?** IF YES: In what way does re-experiencing _(describe flashback)_ influence or control you? (Does the way you _(act, speak, feel, or think)_ remind you of anyone you know or of any past experiences you have had? IF YES: Who does it remind you of? *or* What experience does it remind you of?)	**Influences Actions, Speech, Feelings, Thoughts** ○ Unclear　　○ No　○ Yes　　○ Inconsistent Description:
228. Do you ever talk with yourself (or another person) or have inner dialogues (silently or out loud), when you re-experience _(describe flashback)_**?**	**Inner Talk or Dialogues** ○ Unclear　　○ No　○ Yes　　○ Inconsistent
228a. Have you ever experienced unwanted thoughts or heard voices that you associate with re-experiencing _(describe flashback)_**?** IF YES to 228 or 228a: Can you share an example of what you experienced (or heard)? (How often do you experience _(inner talk, unwanted thoughts, or voices)_ when you relive _(describe flashback)_?)	**Intrusive Thoughts or Voices** ○ Unclear　　○ No　○ Yes　　○ Inconsistent Description:

229. If the part of you that re-experiences $\underline{\hspace{3cm}}$ **could speak, what might that** (describe flashback) **part say?** (What might the part that re-experiences $\underline{\hspace{3cm}}$ say to help us understand more (describe flashback) about $\underline{\hspace{4cm}}$?) (describe flashback, or "you", or "your life")	Description:
If the client's responses suggest an identity disturbance, continue with question 229a. Otherwise, if there are no additional Follow-Up sections you wish to pursue (see page 65), you may end the interview here.	
229a. What does the part of you that re-experiences $\underline{\hspace{3cm}}$ **need to feel more** (describe flashback) **at peace?** (What do you need to feel more at peace with the part of you that re-experiences $\underline{\hspace{3cm}}$?) (describe flashback) *and/or* (What does $\underline{\hspace{5cm}}$ need to ("your adult self" or "your compassionate self") feel more at peace with the part of you that re- experiences $\underline{\hspace{3cm}}$?) (describe flashback)	Description:
*230. Does it feel as if the part of you that re-experiences $\underline{\hspace{3cm}}$ could talk with (describe flashback) a therapist directly? IF YES: Can you describe what might be said?	**Talk With Therapist** ○ Unclear ○ No ○ Yes ○ Inconsistent Description:

231. Does it feel as if the part of you that re-experiences _____ **has different** (describe flashback) **memories, behaviors, feelings, or beliefs than your own, or does it feel similar?** (Or, does it sometimes feel similar and sometimes different?)

   IF DIFFERENT: In what ways are they different?

Different Memories, Behaviors, Feelings, etc.
- ○ unclear
- ○ feels similar
- ○ sometimes feels different
- ○ feels different

Description:

---

232. Does it feel as if the part of you that re-experiences _____ **, is a part of** (describe flashback) **your personality, or does it feel separate?** (Or, does it sometimes feel separate, and sometimes a part of your personality?)

   IF YES (to feels separate): Can you describe what you mean when you say it feels separate?

Separate or Part of Personality
- ○ unclear
- ○ part of personality
- ○ sometimes feels separate, sometimes not
- ○ feels separate

Description:

232a. When you re-experience _____ **,** (describe flashback) **does it feel as if it is happening to you or to someone else?**

   IF YES to feels like it's happening to someone else, ask:
Can you describe what you mean when you say it feels like it's happening to someone else?

Flashback Is Experienced as Self or Other
- ○ unclear
- ○ happening to self
- ○ sometimes feels it's happening to self, sometimes not
- ○ happening to someone else

Description:

233.	**Summary: Personality States** ○ Inadequate information ○ Lacks evidence of 2 or more personality states ○ Suspect 2 or more personality states, but distinctness is unclear ○ Appears to have 2 or more distinct personality states (i.e., with related alterations in affect, memory, behavior, cognition, and/or sensory-motor control)
233a.	**Summary: Shifts in Executive Control/Agency** ○ Inadequate information ○ Lacks evidence of shifts of executive control ○ Shifts in control seem less-than-marked ○ Marked shifts in executive control
If the presence, absence, or type of dissociative disorder is clear, you may end the interview here. If more information is needed, continue with an additional Follow-Up section (see page 65).	

DIFFERENT PERSON FOLLOW-UP

Questions in this follow-up section should be personalized to refer to the "different" person that the client described (characterized by disowned emotions, behaviors, talents, etc.). Examples of personalized fill-in phrases include the "different person," the "third party filled with shame," the "angry, explosive person," "James Bond," the "imposter," etc. This section can be repeated for each "different" person that the interviewer is exploring.

Earlier you mentioned that you have felt as if (or acted as if) you were a different person. Can you say anything more about that? (How do you understand that experience?)	Description:
234. Does it feel as if ——————— **ever** (describe different person) **influences or controls the way you act, speak, feel, or think?** IF YES: In what way does ———————influence or control you? (describe different person) (Does the way you ——————— remind (act, speak, feel, or think) you of anyone you know or of any past experience you have had? IF YES: Who does it remind you of? *or* What experience does it remind you of?)	**Influences Actions, Speech, Feelings, Thoughts** ○ Unclear ○ No ○ Yes ○ Inconsistent Description:
235. Do you have a visual image of ———————? (describe different person) (Do you associate a facial expression, tone of voice, feeling, or movement with ———————?) (describe different person) IF YES: What is the ——————— like? (image, expression, voice, feeling, etc.) (Does the ——————— (image, expression, voice, feeling, etc.) remind you of anyone you know or of any past experience you have had? IF YES: Who does it remind you of? *or* What experience does it remind you of?)	**Image, Voice, Feeling, etc. of Different Person** ○ Unclear ○ No ○ Yes ○ Inconsistent Description:

236. Is there an age (or age range) that you associate with _____? (describe different person)

IF YES: What age or age range?

Age(s) Associated With Person

⊙ Unclear ⊙ No ⊙ Yes ⊙ Inconsistent

Description:

---

237. Is there a name (actual or symbolic) that you associate with _____? (describe different person)

IF YES:
238. What name(s) are you aware of? How did you become aware of this/these name(s)?

Name Associated With Person

⊙ Unclear ⊙ No ⊙ Yes ⊙ Inconsistent

Aware of Name(s)

⊙ unclear
⊙ has 1 or more nicknames or descriptive names
⊙ has 1 other proper name (not nickname)
⊙ has 2–5 other proper names
⊙ has 6 or more proper names

---

239. Have you ever talked with or had inner dialogues with _____ **(silently or out loud)?** (describe different person)

Inner Talk or Dialogues

⊙ Unclear ⊙ No ⊙ Yes ⊙ Inconsistent

239a. Have you ever experienced unwanted thoughts or heard voices that you associate with _____ **?** (describe different person)

IF YES to 239 or 239a: Can you share an example of what was said? (How often do you experience _____ (inner talk, unwanted thoughts, or voices) with _____ ?) (describe different person)

Intrusive Thoughts or Voices

⊙ Unclear ⊙ No ⊙ Yes ⊙ Inconsistent

Description:

240. If _____ **could speak, what**
       (describe different person)

might _____ **say?**
          (describe different person)

(What might _____ say to help us
            (describe different person)

understand more about

_____?)
(describe different person, or "you", or "your life")

Description:

---

*If the client's responses suggest an identity
disturbance, continue with question 240a.
Otherwise, if there are no additional Follow-Up
sections you wish to pursue (see page 65), you
may end the interview here.*

240a. What does _____ **need to**
                    (describe different person)

feel more at peace?

(What do you need to feel more at peace with

_____ ?)
(describe different person)

                    and/or

(What does

_____ need to
("your adult self" or "your compassionate self")

feel more at peace with _____?)
                        (describe different person)

Description:

---

*241. Does it feel as if _____
                            (describe different person)

could talk with a therapist directly?

   IF YES: What might _____
                     (describe different person)

   say?

Talk With a Therapist

○ Unclear   ○ No   ○ Yes   ○ Inconsistent

Description:

---

242. Does it feel as if _____ (describe different person) **has different memories, behaviors, feelings, or beliefs than your own, or does it feel similar?** (Or, does it sometimes feel different and sometimes similar?) IF DIFFERENT: In what way are they different?	**Different Memories, Behaviors, Feelings, etc.** ○ unclear ○ feels similar ○ sometimes feels different ○ feels different Description:
243. Does it feel as if _____ **is** (describe different person) **a part of your personality, or does it feel separate?** (Or, does it sometimes feel separate and sometimes a part of your personality?) IF YES (to feels separate): Can you describe what you mean when you say it feels separate?	**Separate or Part of Personality** ○ unclear ○ part of their personality ○ sometimes feels separate, sometimes not ○ feels separate Description:
244.	**Summary: Personality States** ○ Inadequate information ○ Lacks evidence of 2 or more personality states ○ Suspect 2 or more personality states, but distinctness is unclear ○ Appears to have 2 or more distinct personality states (i.e., with related alterations in affect, memory, behavior, cognition, and/or sensory-motor control)
244a.	**Summary: Shifts in Executive Control/Agency** ○ Inadequate information ○ Lacks evidence of shifts in executive control ○ Shifts in control seem less-than-marked ○ Marked shifts in executive control
If the presence, absence, or type of dissociative disorder is clear, you may end the interview here. If more information is needed, continue with an additional Follow-Up section (see page 65).	

POSSESSION OR TRANCE FOLLOW-UP

Questions should be personalized to refer to the possessing agent or trance state that the client described. Dissociative disorder diagnosis should not be applied to experiences caused by substance use, medical illness, or experiences that are a normal part of an accepted cultural or religious practice. Examples of personalized fill-in phrases for a possessing agent include possessed by "a devil," possessed by "an evil spirit," possessed by "a fox," etc. An example of a possible fill-in phrase for a trance state is having been in a "trance."

Earlier you mentioned that you felt as if you were possessed by _____. (describe possessing agent) *or* **Earlier you mentioned that you had experienced** _____. (describe trance state) **Can you say anything more about that experience?** (How do you understand that experience?) **When you experienced** _____, **were you** (describe possessing agent/trance state) **aware of any changes in how you experienced your surroundings?** IF YES: What changes were you aware of?	*(Common possession states include feeling as if one's behavior or speech is controlled by another person, spirit, supernatural being, or force.)* Description:
If client endorsed feeling possessed, continue with question 245. If client experienced a trance, skip to question 246.	
245. When you felt possessed, did it feel as if _____ **is inside or** (describe possessing agent/trance state) **outside of you?** (Can you say anything more about that experience?)	**Possessed From Inside or Outside** ◯ unclear ◯ possessed from outside ◯ sometimes from outside, sometimes inside ◯ possessed from inside Description:

Cite as: Steinberg M: The SCID-D Interview: Dissociation Assessment in Therapy, Forensics, and Research. Washington, DC, American Psychiatric Association Publishing, 2023

246. Does it feel as if

———————————— **influences or**
(describe possessing agent/ trance state)
controls the way you behave, speak, or move?

(Do you lose control of your behavior or speech

when you feel ————————————?)
(describe possessing agent/trance state)
(Do you experience any unwanted changes in
your behavior, movements, or speech?)

   IF YES: In what way does

   ———————————— influence or
   (describe possessing agent/trance state)
   control you? (What behaviors, speech, or
   movements do you lose control of?) (What type
   of unwanted changes do you experience?)

   (Does the way you ——————— remind
   (act, speak, or move)
   you of anyone you know or of any past
   experiences you have had?)

   IF YES: Who does it remind you of? *or*
   What experience does it remind you of?

Involuntary/Unwanted Changes in Behavior, Speech, or Movements

○ Unclear   ○ No   ○ Yes   ○ Inconsistent

(Common behavioral manifestations associated with feeling possessed include distinct differences in speech or behaviors that feel as if they are outside of the person's control.)

Description:

---

247. Do you have a visual image that you

associate with ————————————?
(describe possessing agent/trance state)
(Do you associate a facial expression, tone of
voice, feeling, or movement with

————————————?)
(describe possessing agent/trance state)

   IF YES: What is the

   ———————————— like?
   (image, expression, voice, feeling, etc.)

   (Does the ————————————
   (image, expression, voice, feeling, etc.)
   remind you of anyone you know, or of any past
   experience you have had?)

   IF YES: Who does it remind you of? *or*
   What experience does it remind you of?

Visual Image of Possessing Agent or Trance

○ Unclear   ○ No   ○ Yes   ○ Inconsistent

Description:

---

248. Is there an age (or age range) that you associate with _____? (describe possessing agent/trance state) IF YES: What age or age range?	**Age(s) Associated With Possession or Trance** ○ Unclear ○ No ○ Yes ○ Inconsistent Description:
249. Do you refer to yourself, or do other people refer to you, by a different name (other than your usual name) when you experience feeling _____? (describe possessing agent/trance state) (When you feel _____, (describe possessing agent/trance state) do you experience any changes or loss in your own identity?) IF YES: **250.** What name(s) are you aware of? (What changes are you aware of in your identity?)	**Different Name or Loss of Identity** ○ Unclear ○ No ○ Yes ○ Inconsistent *(During possession states, the person experiences an alteration in their identity [to that of the possessing agent's identity]. During trance state's [without possession] the person may have a loss of personal identity, without a replacement of identity.)* Description: **Aware of Names** ○ unclear ○ has 1 or more nicknames or descriptive names ○ has 1 other proper name (not nicknames) ○ has 2–5 other proper names ○ has 6 or more proper names ○ experiences a loss of identity
251. Have you ever talked with or had dialogues with _____ (describe possessing agent/trance state) **(silently or out loud)?** (Has _____ ever (describe possessing agent/trance state) talked to you or to other people?)	**Inner Talk or Dialogues** ○ Unclear ○ No ○ Yes ○ Inconsistent

251a. Have you ever experienced unwanted thoughts or heard voices that you associate with _____**?** (describe possessing agent/trance state) IF YES to 251 or 251a: Can you share an example of what _____ says? (describe possessing agent/trance state) (How often do you experience _____ associated (talking, unwanted thoughts, or voices) with _____?) (describe possessing agent/trance state)	**Intrusive Thoughts or Voices** ○ Unclear ○ No ○ Yes ○ Inconsistent Description:
252. If _____ **could** (describe possessing agent/trance state) **speak, what might** _____ **say?** (describe possessing agent/trance state) (What might _____ (describe possessing agent/trance state) say to help us understand more about _____?) (possessing agent/trance state or "you" or "your life")	Description:
If the client's responses suggest an identity disturbance, continue with question 252a. Otherwise, if there are no additional Follow-Up sections you wish to pursue (see page 65), you may end the interview here.	
252a. What does _____ **need to feel** (describe possessing agent/trance state) **more at peace?** (What do you need to feel more at peace with _____?) (describe possessing agent/trance state) *and/or* (What does _____ ("your adult self" or "your compassionate self") need to feel more at peace with _____?) (describe possessing agent/trance state)	Description:

*253. Does it feel as if _____ could talk with (describe possessing agent/trance state) a therapist directly? IF YES: What might _____ say? (describe possessing agent/trance state)	**Talk With Therapist** ○ Unclear ○ No ○ Yes ○ Inconsistent Description:
254. Does it feel as if _____ **has different** (describe possessing agent/trance state) **memories, behaviors, feelings, or beliefs than your own, or does it feel similar?** (Or, does it sometimes feel similar and sometimes different?) IF DIFFERENT: In what way are they different?	**Different Memories, Behaviors, Feelings, etc.** ○ unclear ○ feels similar ○ sometimes feels different ○ feels different Description:
255. Does it feel as if _____ **is a part of** (describe possessing agent/trance state) **your personality, or does it feel separate?** (Or, does it sometimes feel separate and sometimes a part of your personality?) IF YES to feels separate: Can you describe what you mean when you say it feels separate?	**Separate or Part of Personality** ○ unclear ○ part of personality ○ sometimes feels separate, sometimes not ○ feels separate Description:
256. Does your religion, culture, or spiritual interests teach you anything about _____? (describe possessing agent/trance state) IF YES: What does it teach you? (Can you describe your religious beliefs (or practices in your culture) and how it relates to your feeling _____?) (describe possessing agent/trance state)	**Religious/Culturally Accepted Possession or Trance** ○ Unclear ○ No ○ Yes ○ Inconsistent Description:

256a. When you experience feeling _____, **does that** (describe possessing agent/trance state) **interfere with your social relationships or affect your ability to function?** IF YES: How does it interfere with your relationships (or ability to function)?	**Interferes With Functioning** ○ Unclear ○ No ○ Yes ○ Inconsistent Description:
256b. When you experience feeling _____, **does that** (describe possessing agent/trance state) **cause you discomfort (or distress)?** IF YES: Can you describe your discomfort or distress?	**Discomfort or Distress** ○ unclear ○ does not cause distress ○ sometimes causes distress ○ usually causes distress Description:
257. *(Rate the possession or trance state within the client's religious or cultural context.)*	**Possession or Trance: Cultural Context** ○ unclear ○ appears normative within culture ○ does not appear normative within culture
258.	**Summary: Personality States** ○ Inadequate information ○ Lacks evidence of 2 or more personality states ○ Suspect 2 or more personality states, but distinctness is unclear ○ Appears to have 2 or more distinct personality states (i.e., with related alterations in affect, memory, behavior, cognition, and/or sensory-motor control)
258a.	**Summary: Shifts in Executive Control/Agency** ○ Inadequate information ○ Lacks evidence of shifts in executive control ○ Shifts in control seem less-than-marked ○ Marked shifts in executive control
If the presence, absence, or type of dissociative disorder is clear, you may end the interview here. If more information is needed, continue with an additional Follow-Up section (see page 65).	

ICD-11-Specific Follow-Up: DID versus Partial DID

This follow-up section has been added to the SCID-D for exploring the new ICD classification of Partial DID. This section may be useful for researchers investigating whether Partial DID is meaningfully distinct from DID, and if so, how it may differ. If the client's responses indicate the presence or experience of "two or more distinct personality states (dissociative identities), involving discontinuities in the sense of self and agency," and it is unclear whether the criteria for ICD-11's DID versus Partial DID are met, ask the questions in this section (questions 258.01–258.12). This section can be repeated for each personality state that intrudes and is under review.

Dr. Steinberg is grateful for the contributions of Dr. Olivier Piedfort-Marin for his recommendations regarding questions in this ICD-11 Specific Follow-Up section.

You've described having more than one personality state. I'll now ask you about each personality's role in your daily functioning, such as work and parenting.	*(In Partial DID, one distinct personality state is dominant and functions in daily life. In DID, two or more distinct personality states recurrently take executive control of daily functioning [e.g., parenting or work].)*
258.01 Does it feel as if one personality state, or more than one (personality state), controls your daily functioning?	**Number of Personality States That Control Daily Functioning** ○ Unclear ○ Only one personality state controls daily functioning ○ Two or more personality states control daily functioning ○ Inconsistent information
If one personality state controls daily functioning, skip to question 258.04 on page 112. *If two or more personality states control daily functioning, continue with question 258.02.*	
258.02 Which personality states control your daily functioning?	Description:
258.03 Can you describe the daily functions that are performed by each personality state?	Description:

If it's clear that two or more distinct personality states control daily functioning, you may end the interview here and then rate the Nonverbal/ Observable Cues (starting on page 119).	
258.04 Which personality state controls your daily functioning?	**One Personality State is Dominant and Controls Functioning** Description:
258.05 Can you describe the daily functions that are performed when —————————————— **is in control of** (describe dominant personality state) **your functioning?**	**Daily Functions of Dominant Personality** Description:
258.06 Do you experience any personality states that influence (or interfere with) your daily functioning? IF YES: Continue with 258.07 IF NO: You may conclude your interview here, and then rate the Nonverbal/Observable Cues (starting on page 119).	**Nondominant Personality States Intrude on Functioning** O Unclear O No O Yes O Inconsistent information Description:
258.07 Which personality states influence (or interfere with) your functioning?	Description:
258.08 Can you describe how —————————————— **influences** (describe nondominant personality state) **(or interferes with) your functioning?**	Description:

258.09 Can you describe the type of situations that might result in _____ **influencing** (describe nondominant personality state) **(or interfering with) your daily functioning?**	*(In Partial DID, the nondominant personality states do not recurrently take executive control of the individual's consciousness and functioning to the extent that they perform in specific aspects of daily life [e.g., parenting, work]. However, there may be occasional, limited, and transient episodes in which a distinct personality state assumes executive control to engage in circumscribed behaviors [e.g., in response to extreme emotional states, during episodes of self-harm, or the reenactment of traumatic memories].)* Description:
258.10 What makes you aware that _____ **is** (describe nondominant personality state) **influencing (or interfering with) your functioning?**	Description:
258.11 How often does _____ **influence** (describe nondominant personality state) **(or interfere with) your functioning?**	**Frequency of Intrusions** ○ unclear ○ rarely (up to 4 isolated episodes) ○ occasionally (up to 4 episodes per year) ○ frequently (5 or more episodes per year) ○ monthly (up to 3 episodes per month) ○ daily/weekly (4 or more episodes per month)
258.12 Does it cause you distress when _____ **influences** (describe nondominant personality state) **(or interferes with) your functioning?** IF YES: How distressing is it?	**Intrusions Cause Distress** ○ Unclear ○ No ○ Yes ○ Inconsistent Description:
If the presence, absence, or type of dissociative disorder is clear, you may end the interview here. Otherwise, consider administering an additional Follow-Up section (see page 65).	

DSM-5-TR SPECIFIC: OPTIONAL HISTORY QUESTIONS
RELEVANT TO OTHER SPECIFIED DISSOCIATIVE DISORDER (OSDD), EXAMPLE 2

Note: Questions in this section should be asked only if OSDD is the likely diagnosis, and it is unclear which OSDD dissociative symptom example type the person suffers from. The questions in this section ask about traumatic life experiences associated with OSDD Example 2 (Identity disturbance due to prolonged and intense coercive persuasion) and may be triggering to trauma survivors; if you elect to pursue questions H40 through H42, please allow sufficient time to sensitively ask and reply to a client's responses. Unless there is a need to distinguish OSDD Example 2 from other OSDD examples, the questions on this page can be skipped.

Past Stressors	
H40. Have you ever been subjected to prolonged brainwashing, for example by a sect or cult or other organization? IF YES: Can you describe what you experienced? How old were you when you experienced _____? (client's endorsed experience) (How long did you experience _____? (client's endorsed experience) How has this experience affected your life?)	**Coercive Influence** ○ Unclear ○ No ○ Yes Description:
H41. Have you ever been kidnapped or otherwise held captive? IF YES: Can you describe what occurred? How old were you when you experienced _____? (client's endorsed experience) (How long were you _____? (client's endorsed experience) How has this experience affected your life?)	**Kidnapped or Held Captive** ○ Unclear ○ No ○ Yes Description:
H42. Have you ever been a political prisoner or been tortured? IF YES: Can you describe what occurred? How old were you when you experienced _____? (client's endorsed experience) (How long were you _____? (client's endorsed experience) How has this experience affected your life?)	**Political Prisoner or Tortured** ○ Unclear ○ No ○ Yes Description:

PART IV:
POST-INTERVIEW RATINGS

NONVERBAL/OBSERVABLE CUES

(Observed During the Interview)

This section lists various nonverbal/observable cues that can occur in people suffering from dissociative experiences. One or more of these symptoms may have been observed *during* the interview itself and should be rated *after* the interview has been completed. The presence of any of these nonverbal cues, in the context of clinically significant dissociative symptoms, can provide additional evidence in support of a dissociative disorder diagnosis.

259. Alteration in client's demeanor. *(Distinct changes in emotional or voice tone, behavior, body movements, or general style of responding. Example: Client switches from a calm, cooperative, articulate individual to an anxious, fearful, paranoid person. There is no clear cause of this change.)*	**Alteration of Demeanor** ○ Unclear ○ No ○ Yes ○ Inconsistent Description:
259a. Movement disturbance. *(Unwanted movements, including tremor, shaking, tics, pseudoseizures, gait abnormality, etc., without known medical origin.)*	**Movement Disturbance** ○ Unclear ○ No ○ Yes ○ Inconsistent Description:
259b. Paralysis or muscle weakness. *(Paralysis [part or all of a limb], difficulty intentionally moving parts of the body, etc., without known medical origin.)*	**Paralysis or Weakness** ○ Unclear ○ No ○ Yes ○ Inconsistent Description:
259c. Speech disturbance. *(Speech impairment, difficulty speaking, muteness, etc., without known medical origin.)*	**Speech Disturbance** ○ Unclear ○ No ○ Yes ○ Inconsistent Description:
259d. Sensory disturbance. *(Loss or disturbed vision, hearing, or loss [partial or complete] of any sensation [e.g., touch, pin prick, vibration, heat, cold] without known medical origin.)*	**Sensory Disturbance** ○ Unclear ○ No ○ Yes ○ Inconsistent Description:

Cite as: Steinberg M: The SCID-D Interview: Dissociation Assessment in Therapy, Forensics, and Research. Washington, DC, American Psychiatric Association Publishing, 2023

259e. Impaired cognitive performance in memory, language, or other cognitive domains. *(Symptoms are not consistent with a medical/ neuro-logical disorder, or due to substance use.)*	**Impaired Cognition** ○ Unclear ○ No ○ Yes ○ Inconsistent Description:
260. Alteration in client's identity. *(Client experiences an alteration in their usual sense of personal identity. The new identity is attributed to the influence of another personality state, spirit, power, or deity.)*	**Alteration of Identity** ○ Unclear ○ No ○ Yes ○ Inconsistent Description:
261. Spontaneous age regression or childlike behavior in an adult. *(Age regression involves "reliving the past as though it were occurring in the present, with age-appropriate vocabulary, mental content, and affect" (Spiegel and Rosenfeld 1984, p. 522). Example: Client switches from sitting and responding calmly to a childlike demeanor squirming in the chair and sucking her thumb.)*	**Age Regression** ○ Unclear ○ No ○ Yes ○ Inconsistent Description:
262. Inconsistencies/fluctuations in level of function and/or mood. *(Example: Client is calm, mature, articulate, and intelligent yet experiences difficulty understanding numerous interview questions and intermittently has difficulty responding to some of the questions.)*	**Fluctuations in Mood and Functioning** ○ Unclear ○ No ○ Yes ○ Inconsistent Description:
263. Client refers to themself in the first-person plural ("we") or third person ("he/she/they").	**Self-reference** ○ Unclear ○ No ○ Yes ○ Inconsistent Description:
264. Client is noted to talk to themself or reports intra-interview internal dialogues (or voices), although they are not psychotic.	**Talks to Self** ○ Unclear ○ No ○ Yes ○ Inconsistent Description:

265. Intra-interview amnesia (Kluft 1985). *(Example 1: Client repeatedly forgets what they were talking about or what the interviewer asked.)*	**Intra-interview Amnesia** ○ Unclear ○ No ○ Yes ○ Inconsistent Description:
266. Intra-interview depersonalization. *(Client remarks during the interview that they feel disconnected or unreal [e.g., their "real" self is far away or that they can see themselves from a distance].)*	**Intra-interview Depersonalization** ○ Unclear ○ No ○ Yes ○ Inconsistent Description:
267. Intra-interview derealization. *(Client remarks during the interview that they feel that the environment [i.e., the interview, the interviewer, or the room] feels as if it is unreal.)*	**Intra-interview Derealization** ○ Unclear ○ No ○ Yes ○ Inconsistent Description:
268. Responses such as "I don't know" or "I don't remember" to questions that appear basic, in a client who appears cooperative and genuinely puzzled.	**Confusion Regarding Responses** ○ Unclear ○ No ○ Yes ○ Inconsistent Description:
269. Ambivalent or inconsistent responses regarding dissociative symptoms. *(Client responds in both the positive and negative or responds in a vague manner that could be interpreted as either yes or no. Example 1: Client responds "yes" to a question and simultaneously shakes his head from side to side, suggesting "no." Example 2: Client responds with a muffled utterance that sounds slightly like "yes" and slightly like "no." Example 3: Client exhibits lengthy pauses prior to responding and then answers "no" or evades the question.)*	**Ambivalent Responses** ○ Unclear ○ No ○ Yes ○ Inconsistent Description:
270. Significant emotional response to SCID-D questions regarding dissociative symptoms. *(Emotional responses seem out of proportion to the question [e.g., heavy sighs, inappropriate laughter, long pauses, or numerous requests to repeat questions and/or skip questions].)*	**Emotional Responses** ○ Unclear ○ No ○ Yes ○ Inconsistent Description:

271. Eye movements suggestive of hypnotic state (in the absence of ocular or neurological disease). *(Movements may include lid fluttering, eyes rolling upward, eyes moving rapidly from side-to-side, and/or eyes closed for prolonged periods during the interview.)*	**Auto-Hypnotic State** ○ Unclear ○ No ○ Yes ○ Inconsistent Description:
272. Trance-like state/narrowing of awareness of one's surroundings. *(Trance is characterized by a marked alteration in one's state of consciousness. This may include loss of one's customary sense of personal identity, narrowing of one's awareness of one's environment, or limitation of one's movements, postures, or speech. The client may exhibit a blank stare or slowed movements or speech.)*	**Trancelike State** ○ Unclear ○ No ○ Yes ○ Inconsistent Description:

APPENDIX 1:
SCID-D SEVERITY RATING DEFINITIONS

SEVERITY RATING DEFINITIONS
OF AMNESIA SYMPTOMS

AMNESIA (DISSOCIATIVE) – A subjective sense of gaps in one's memory for autobiographical information or experiences, or for blocks of time that have passed, where such lapses cannot be attributed to ordinary forgetfulness. Amnesia is clinically significant if it results in dysfunction and/or significant distress.	**SCID-D Items**
MILD (SUBCLINICAL)	
Frequency and Qualitative Cues:	
Transient forgetfulness of a minor nature (i.e., forgetting where you placed your keys or glasses), or amnesia limited to one's very early childhood.	1–36
Mild amnesia typically exhibits the following quality:	
• The person is usually able to soon recall the minor events that were initially forgotten.	22
The memory lapses must meet both of the following:	
• Does not cause impairment in social, occupational, or other important functioning.	21
• Does not cause significant distress.	23
MODERATE (CLINICALLY SIGNIFICANT)	
Frequency and Qualitative Cues:	
Memory gaps or problems in one's memory occur once per month or less frequently. The memory gaps cannot be attributed to ordinary forgetfulness.	1–36
Moderate amnesia typically exhibits one or more of the following qualities:	
• Recurrent brief amnestic episodes (if prolonged amnesia, rate as severe).	1–20
• Frequent difficulty with memory, or recalling personal events or time periods.	1–20
• Episodes of amnesia, loss of time, "blank spells" lasting no more than several hours.	1–20
• Client is unable to report the frequency of their amnestic episodes or appears puzzled or confused as to the frequency.	1–20
• Episodes of amnesia (four or fewer) not precipitated by stress.	22
• Prolonged episodes of amnesia (four or fewer) (lasting over 4 hours).	3–5
• Amnesia may be triggered by substance use but also occurs without substance use.	24–25
Intra-Interview Cues (may exhibit the following):	
• Up to two "blank spells" or brief amnestic episodes during interview.	265
The memory lapses must meet one or both of the following:	
• Causes impairment in social, occupational, or other important functioning.	21
• Causes significant distress.	23

The Severity Rating Definitions are not an inclusive list. The purpose of these definitions is to give the rater a general description of the parameters of the spectrum of dissociative symptoms and their severity.

Cite as: Steinberg M: The SCID-D Interview: Dissociation Assessment in Therapy, Forensics, and Research. Washington, DC, American Psychiatric Association Publishing, 2023

SEVERE (CLINICALLY SIGNIFICANT)	
Frequency and Qualitative Cues:	
Recurrent to ongoing memory problems or gaps in one's memory (more frequent than once a month, e.g., weekly, daily, or persistent) that cannot be attributed to ordinary forgetfulness. Common manifestations include recurrently experiencing memory lapses, difficulty recalling significant events or time periods, or the sense that time is missing or is discontinuous.	1–36
Severe amnesia typically exhibits one or more of the following qualities:	
• Prolonged episodes of amnesia (five or more, lasting four hours or longer).	1–20
• Recurrent memory gaps, (brief or prolonged) or the sense that time feels discontinuous, most of the time.	1–20
• Finding oneself in a place away from home, unaware of how or why they went there, or with amnesia for autobiographical information.	7–14
• Large memory gap(s) for significant autobiographical events or for blocks of time after very early childhood.	1–20
• Unable to remember one's name, age, address, or other personal information.	9–16
• Describes abilities and/or talents that they cannot recall learning or has episodes of "forgetting" acquired skills (e.g., a skilled chef states that they "forgot" how to cook).	1–21, 135
• Other people report that the client is experiencing memory problems or gaps in memory (that cannot be attributed to substance use or medical illness).	1–21
• Amnesia may be triggered by stress but often occurs without stress.	22
• Amnesia may be triggered by substance use but also occurs without substance use.	24–25
• Clients with long-standing amnesia for specific significant autobiographical events or time periods may not report distress associated with their amnesia, preferring "not to know." In such cases, clients may experience increased dysfunction and/or distress when they begin to regain information from their amnestic time periods.	21–23
Intra-Interview Cues (may exhibit the following):	
• Significant intra-interview amnesia (e.g., experiences repeated episodes of amnesia during interview, becomes disoriented, or unaware of who they are or who interviewer is).	Full SCID-D
The memory lapses must meet one or both of the following:	
• Causes impairment in social, occupational, or other important functioning	21
• Causes significant distress.	23

SEVERITY RATING DEFINITIONS
OF DEPERSONALIZATION SYMPTOMS

DEPERSONALIZATION (DP)—A feeling of disconnection from one's self (e.g., from one's feelings, thoughts, behavior, or body), or a sense of being an outside observer of one's self. DP is clinically significant if it results in dysfunction and/or significant distress.	SCID-D Items
MILD (SUBCLINICAL)	
Frequency and Qualitative Cues:	
Single or few episodes of DP (1–4 episodes) that are typically transient.	38–48, 55–62
Mild DP typically exhibits one or more of the following qualities:	
• The DP is usually brief and lasts less than 4 hours.	55–61
• The DP is commonly triggered by severe stress, acute trauma, or substance use.	64, 72–74
• The DP may be triggered by an adverse effect of medication, exhaustion, sensory deprivation, or hypnagogic/hypnopompic states.	72–75
Mild DP must meet both of the following:	
• Does not cause impairment in social, occupational, or other important functioning.	63
• Does not cause significant distress.	65
MODERATE (CLINICALLY SIGNIFICANT)	
Frequency and Qualitative Cues:	
DP episodes occur once per month or less frequently. Common manifestations include feeling detached, estranged, unreal, numb, and/or like an observer of oneself.	38–62
Moderate DP typically exhibits one or more of the following qualities:	
• The duration of a DP episode typically lasts less than 24 hours.	55
• DP may be triggered by stress but also occurs without stress.	64
• DP may be triggered by substance use but also occurs without substance use.	72–73
• The intensity and nature of DP symptoms may vary over time.	38–62
Moderate DP must meet one or both of the following:	
• Causes impairment in social, occupational, or other important functioning.	63
• Causes significant distress.	65

The Severity Rating Definitions are not an inclusive list. The purpose of these definitions is to give the rater a general description of the parameters of the spectrum of dissociative symptoms and their severity.

Cite as: Steinberg M: The SCID-D Interview: Dissociation Assessment in Therapy, Forensics, and Research. Washington, DC, American Psychiatric Association Publishing, 2023

SEVERE (CLINICALLY SIGNIFICANT)	
Frequency and Qualitative Cues:	
Recurrent to ongoing DP (more frequent than once a month [e.g., weekly, daily, or persistent]). Common manifestations include feeling detached, estranged, unreal, numb, and/or like an observer of one's self.	38–62
Severe DP typically exhibits one or more of the following qualities:	
• Severe DP may manifest as feeling like a stranger to oneself, feeling as if one is losing one's sense of identity, feeling invisible, or having difficulty recognizing oneself in a mirror.	40, 43
• DP questions elicit spontaneous descriptions of interactive dialogues between observing and participating self.	38–53
• DP questions elicit spontaneous descriptions of identity confusion or alteration.	38–53
• The duration of a DP episode may last longer than 24 hours.	55
• DP may be triggered by stress but also occurs without stress.	64
• DP may be triggered by substance use but also occurs without substance use.	72–73
• The intensity and nature of DP symptoms may vary over time.	38–62
• Clients with long-standing severe DP may not report distress because of acclimation to the DP.	65
Severe DP must meet one or both of the following:	
• Causes impairment in social, occupational, or other important functioning.	63
• Causes significant distress.	65

SEVERITY RATING DEFINITIONS
OF DEREALIZATION SYMPTOMS

DEREALIZATION (DR)—A feeling of disconnection from one's surroundings (e.g., people or surroundings feel as if they are unfamiliar, unreal, or distorted). DR is clinically significant if it results in dysfunction and/or significant distress.	SCID-D Items
MILD (SUBCLINICAL)	
Frequency and Qualitative Cues:	
Single or few episodes of DR (1–4 episodes) that are typically transient.	79–93
Mild DR typically exhibits one or more of the following qualities:	
• The DR is usually brief and lasts less than 4 hours.	86
• The DR is commonly triggered by severe stress, acute trauma, or substance use.	92, 95–97
• The DR may be triggered by exhaustion, sensory deprivation, or hypnagogic/hypnopompic states.	98
Mild DR must meet both of the following:	
• Does not cause impairment in social, occupational, or other important functioning.	91
• Does not cause significant distress.	93
MODERATE (CLINICALLY SIGNIFICANT)	
Frequency and Qualitative Cues:	
DR episodes occur once per month or less frequently. Common manifestations include feeling emotionally disconnected from familiar people or surroundings, feelings one's surroundings are dream-like, and/or experiencing perceptual distortions with respect to one's surroundings.	79–93
Moderate DR typically exhibits one or more of the following qualities:	
• The duration of a DR episode typically lasts less than 24 hours.	86
• DR may be triggered by stress but also occurs without stress.	92
• DR may be triggered by substance use but also occurs without substance use.	95–96
• The intensity and nature of DR symptoms may vary over time.	79–84
Moderate DR must meet one or both of the following:	
• Causes impairment in social, occupational, or other important functioning.	91
• Causes significant distress.	93

The Severity Rating Definitions are not an inclusive list. The purpose of these definitions is to give the rater a general description of the parameters of the spectrum of dissociative symptoms and their severity.

Cite as: Steinberg M: The SCID-D Interview: Dissociation Assessment in Therapy, Forensics, and Research. Washington, DC, American Psychiatric Association Publishing, 2023

SEVERE (CLINICALLY SIGNIFICANT)	
Frequency and Qualitative Cues:	
Recurrent to ongoing DR (more frequent than once a month [e.g., weekly, daily, or persistent]). Common manifestations include feeling emotionally disconnected from familiar people or surroundings, feelings one's surroundings are dreamlike, and/or experiencing perceptual distortions with respect to one's surroundings.	79–93
Severe DR typically exhibits one or more of the following qualities:	
• DR may be triggered by stress but also occurs without stress.	92
• Difficulty recognizing close friends, family, or one's home.	82
• The duration of a DR episode can last longer than 24 hours.	86
• DR may be triggered by substance use but also occurs without substance use.	95–96
• The intensity and nature of DR symptoms may vary over time.	79–84
Severe DR must meet one or both of the following:	
• Causes impairment in social, occupational, or other important functioning.	91
• Causes significant distress.	93

SEVERITY RATING DEFINITIONS
OF IDENTITY CONFUSION SYMPTOMS

IDENTITY CONFUSION—Subjective feelings of uncertainty, puzzlement, conflict, or struggle regarding one's own identity or sense of self. Identity confusion is clinically significant if it results in dysfunction and/or significant distress.	SCID-D Items
MILD (SUBCLINICAL)	
Frequency and Qualitative Cues:	
Single or few episodes of confusion, uncertainty, conflict as to one's own identity/sense of self. Mild identity confusion is often associated with conflicts or uncertainty about one's goals, life purpose, or how best to balance one's various social roles (e.g., mother, wife, engineer).	101–112
Common manifestations of mild identity confusion include (all of the following):	
• Adolescents and young adults commonly express confusion about their career choice, educational plans, and life goals.	101–105
• Mild identity confusion is commonly triggered by severe stress, loss, or life transitions.	101–112
• Mild identity confusion usually lasts for a limited period of time.	106–108
• There are no memory gaps related to one's identity and behavior.	1–23, 101–131
• Identity is continuous over time and place.	1–23, 101–131
Mild identity confusion must meet both of the following:	
• Does not cause impairment in social, occupational, or other important functioning.	110
• Does not cause significant distress.	112
MODERATE (CLINICALLY SIGNIFICANT)	
Frequency and Qualitative Cues:	
Identity confusion occurs once per month or less frequently and is characterized by feelings of uncertainty, puzzlement, conflict, or inner struggle as to one's identity.	101–112
Moderate identity confusion typically exhibits one or more of the following qualities:	
• Feeling as if there are different parts/sides of one's personality in conflict with each another.	101–105, 159–169
• Feeling as if one has a childlike and/or critical part of self.	105–112
• Recurrent internal interactive dialogues or voices that criticize self and/or other people, or hearing voices of a child. The critical dialogues or voices may be alternatively described as intrusive thoughts.	138–156
• The intensity and nature of the identity confusion may vary over time.	101–112
• May be triggered by stress, but also occurs without stress.	111

The Severity Rating Definitions are not an inclusive list. The purpose of these definitions is to give the rater a general description of the parameters of the spectrum of dissociative symptoms and their severity.

Cite as: Steinberg M: The SCID-D Interview: Dissociation Assessment in Therapy, Forensics, and Research. Washington, DC, American Psychiatric Association Publishing, 2023

Moderate identity confusion must meet one or both of the following:	
• Causes impairment in social, occupational, or other important functioning.	110
• Causes significant distress.	112
SEVERE (CLINICALLY SIGNIFICANT)	
Frequency and Qualitative Cues:	
Recurrent to ongoing episodes of identity confusion (more frequent than once a month [e.g., weekly, daily, or persistent]), characterized by recurrent feelings of uncertainty, puzzlement, conflict, or inner struggle as to one's identity.	101–112
Severe identity confusion typically exhibits one or more of the following qualities:	
• Feeling as if there are different parts or sides of one's personality in conflict with one another.	101–105
• Feeling as if one has a childlike and/or critical part of self.	105b–e, 113, 138a,b
• Recurrent internal interactive dialogues or voices that criticize self and/or other people, or hearing voices of a child. The critical dialogues or voices may be alternatively described as intrusive thoughts.	138–156
• Significant conflict, struggles, or confusion with respect to basic preferences and seemingly simple decisions.	101–108
• A subjective sense of loss of one's identity.	11, 102–105,
• The intensity and nature of the identity confusion may vary over time.	101–112
Severe identity confusion must meet one or both of the following:	
• Causes impairment in social, occupational, or other important functioning.	110
• Causes significant distress.	112

SEVERITY RATING DEFINITIONS
OF IDENTITY ALTERATION SYMPTOMS

IDENTITY ALTERATION (IA)—Observable behavior associated with alterations or shifts in one's identity or personality states. Identity alteration is clinically significant if there is evidence of personality states, and/or shifts in executive control/agency, and the identity alteration results in dysfunction and/or significant distress.	SCID-D Items
MILD (SUBCLINICAL)	
Qualitative Cues	
Shifts in mood or behavior corresponding to various social roles (e.g. mother, wife, engineer) and/or situational changes. The shifts in mood and behavior must meet <u>all</u> of the following:	113–158
• Does not cause impairment in social, occupational, or other important functioning.	129
• Does not cause significant distress.	131
• No evidence that the client lacks control of their mood or behavior.	113–158
• No evidence of amnesia with respect to shifts in mood, behavior, or social role changes.	1–18, 113–135
MODERATE (CLINICALLY SIGNIFICANT)	
Frequency and Qualitative Cues:	
Recurrent instances of less-than-marked shifts in executive control/agency, and/or the presence of less-than-distinct personality states. Typically these shifts/state-changes are characterized by subtle and/or puzzling fluctuations in mood and/or behavior (e.g., level of functioning or capabilities).	113–158, Follow-Up Sections
Moderate identity alteration typically exhibits one or more of the following qualities:	
• Inner dialogues or hearing voices occurs in the context of less-than-distinct personality states.	138–158, 202–211
• The less-than-distinct personality states do not experience different memories.	159–258
• Episodes of possession in the absence of dissociative amnesia.	1–23, 124–127, 245–258
• The possessing agent appears to be a less-than-distinct personality state.	245–258
• Dissociative trance as evidenced by severe unresponsiveness or insensitivity to one's environment (not part of a broadly accepted cultural or religious practice).	Full SCID-D
• The intensity and nature of the identity alteration may vary over time.	113–158
Intra-Interview Cues (may exhibit one or more of the following):	
• Subtle changes in voice, speech, behavior, demeanor, movement characteristics, or general style of response corresponding to less-than-marked shifts in executive control and/or less-than-distinct personality state.	Full SCID-D

The Severity Rating Definitions are not an inclusive list. The purpose of these definitions is to give the rater a general description of the parameters of the spectrum of dissociative symptoms and their severity.

Cite as: Steinberg M: The SCID-D Interview: Dissociation Assessment in Therapy, Forensics, and Research. Washington, DC, American Psychiatric Association Publishing, 2023

Moderate identity alteration must meet one or both of the following:	
• Causes impairment in social, occupational, or other important functioning.	129
• Causes significant distress.	131
SEVERE (CLINICALLY SIGNIFICANT)	
Frequency and Qualitative Cues:	
Recurrent instances of marked shifts in executive control/agency, and/or the presence of distinct personality states. Typically these shifts/state-changes are characterized by distinct and/or contradictory fluctuations in mood and/or behavior (e.g., level of functioning or capabilities).	113–158, Follow-Up Sections
Severe identity alteration typically exhibits one or more of the following qualities:	
• Amnesia/memory lapses for shifts in one's mood or behavior.	1–23,113–258
• Inner dialogues or hearing voices occur in the context of distinct personality states, associated with different memories, behaviors, or feelings.	138–258
• The distinct personality states experience different memories.	159–258
• Regressed behavior, acting like a child or a different person	113–258
• Childlike part or other personality state feels as if it is separate (i.e., not part of their personality).	159–258
• Feeling as if one is possessed by another person, spirit, supernatural being, or force. The possessing agent appears to be a distinct personality state and occurs in a client who also experiences dissociative amnesia.	1–23,124–127, 245–258
• The use of different names (without apparent secondary gain).	118–121
• Evidence of inconsistent and/or puzzling beliefs and/or ethics resulting in unstable, unpredictable, and/or contradictory behaviors.	Full SCID-D
• Recurrent episodes of finding belongings in one's possession that are inconsistent with one's preferences and/or one could not recall acquiring.	1–23,122–123
• The intensity and nature of the identity alteration may vary over time.	113–158
Intra-interview Cues (may exhibit one or more of the following):	
• Overt changes in voice, speech, behavior, demeanor, movement characteristics, or general style of response corresponding to marked shifts in executive control and/or distinct personality state.	Full SCID-D
• Contradictory responses to questions (e.g., verbally says "yes" while shaking their head from side to side as if to indicate "no").	Full SCID-D
• Recurrent spontaneous reference to self in first-person plural or third person.	Full SCID-D
Severe identity alteration must meet one or both of the following:	
• Causes impairment in social, occupational, or other important functioning.	129
• Causes significant distress.	131

APPENDIX 2:
TYPICAL SCID-D SYMPTOM PROFILES FOR THE DISSOCIATIVE DISORDERS

TYPICAL SCID-D SYMPTOM PROFILES FOR THE DISSOCIATIVE DISORDERS

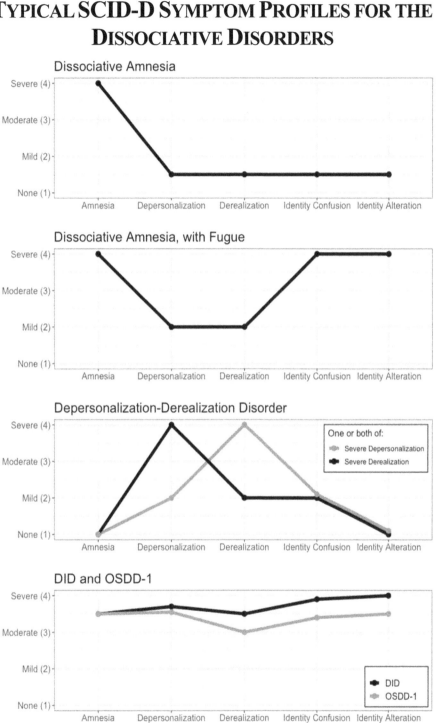

OSDD-1 includes "chronic and recurrent syndromes of mixed dissociative symptoms." OSDD-1 includes "identity disturbance associated with less-than-marked discontinuities in sense of self and agency" (DSM-5-TR).

Figure is adapted with permission from Steinberg M.: *Handbook for the Assessment of Dissociation: A Clinical Guide*. Washington, DC, American Psychiatric Press, 1995.

Cite as: Steinberg M: The SCID-D Interview: Dissociation Assessment in Therapy, Forensics, and Research. Washington, DC, American Psychiatric Association Publishing, 2023

APPENDIX 3A:
ICD-11 DIAGNOSTIC CRITERIA
FOR THE DISSOCIATIVE DISORDERS

ICD-11 DIAGNOSTIC CRITERIA (ESSENTIAL FEATURES) FOR THE DISSOCIATIVE DISORDERS

The information gleaned in the SCID-D interview can be used to determine which ICD dissociative disorder criteria have been fulfilled, and consequently which particular Dissociative Disorder diagnosis, if any, is present. Table 1 below lists the various dissociative disorders classified in ICD-11, along with the page numbers which list the corresponding ICD criteria.

Before considering the ICD essential features, it is often helpful to first complete Section A of the *SCID-D Summary Scoresheet* (see Appendix 4A, page 159), which rates the severity of each of the five SCID-D symptoms. Completing that section of the *Scoresheet* beforehand will inform the likely ICD diagnosis (e.g., by identifying whether moderate-to-severe levels of amnesia co-occur with high levels of several other SCID-D symptoms, suggesting a DID or Partial DID diagnosis, or alternatively if amnesia is the only elevated symptom, suggesting a Dissociative Amnesia diagnosis). It is also helpful, before considering the ICD essential features, to compare your client's SCID-D symptom severity scores to profile norms of research participants with confirmed dissociative disorders (see Appendix 4C, page 167 for a graphical representation of averaged profiles of SCID-D symptom severity scores for previous research participants with confirmed DID or OSDD (née DDNOS) diagnosis). For further discussion of the dissociative symptom profiles for each of the dissociative disorders, see the *Interviewer's Guide to the SCID-D*.

After completing the dissociative symptoms severity on the *SCID-D Summary Scoresheet*, select the ICD dissociative disorder in Table 1 that you believe the client has, refer to the corresponding page mentioned in the table, and rate the presence or absence of the specific diagnostic features to determine if the client's presentation meets the criteria listed.

Table 1: Diagnosing Dissociative Disorders Based on ICD-11

Dissociative Disorder	ICD-11 Essential Features
Dissociative Amnesia	page 142
Depersonalization-Derealization Disorder	page 143
Dissociative Identity Disorder	page 144
Partial Dissociative Identity Disorder	page 145
Other Specified Dissociative Disorder	page 146
Trance Disorder	page 147
Possession Trance Disorder	page 148
Dissociative Neurological Symptom Disorder	pages 149–150

ICD-11 DISSOCIATIVE AMNESIA: ESSENTIAL FEATURES

Dissociative Amnesia, 1ˢᵗ Essential Feature   ◯ Unclear   ◯ No   ◯ Yes
Inability to recall important autobiographical memories, typically of recent traumatic or stressful events, that is inconsistent with ordinary forgetting.

Dissociative Amnesia, 2ⁿᵈ Essential Feature   ◯ Unclear   ◯ No   ◯ Yes
The memory loss does not occur exclusively during episodes of Trance Disorder, Possession Trance Disorder, Dissociative Identity Disorder, or Partial Dissociative Identity Disorder and is not better accounted for by another mental disorder (e.g., Post-Traumatic Stress Disorder, Complex Post-Traumatic Stress Disorder, a Neurocognitive Disorder such as Dementia).

Dissociative Amnesia, 3ʳᵈ Essential Feature   ◯ Unclear   ◯ No   ◯ Yes
The symptoms are not due to the effect of a substance or medication on the central nervous system (e.g., alcohol), including withdrawal effects, and are not due to a Disease of the Nervous System (e.g., temporal lobe epilepsy), another medical condition (e.g., a brain tumor) or to head trauma.

Dissociative Amnesia, 4ᵗʰ Essential Feature   ◯ Unclear   ◯ No   ◯ Yes
The memory loss results in significant impairment in personal, family, social, educational, occupational or other important areas of functioning.

Presence or absence of dissociative fugue:

- **Dissociative Amnesia with dissociative fugue**   ◯ Unclear   ◯ No   ◯ Yes
Dissociative Amnesia with dissociative fugue is characterized by all of the features of Dissociative Amnesia, accompanied by dissociative fugue, i.e., a loss of a sense of personal identity and sudden travel away from home, work, or significant others for an extended period of time (days or weeks).

- **Dissociative Amnesia without dissociative fugue**   ◯ Unclear   ◯ No   ◯ Yes
Dissociative Amnesia without dissociative fugue is characterized by all of the features of Dissociative Amnesia occurring in the absence of symptoms of dissociative fugue.

ICD-11 DEPERSONALIZATION-DEREALIZATION (DP-DR) DISORDER: ESSENTIAL FEATURES

DP-DR Disorder, 1st Essential Feature　　　　○ Unclear　　○ No　　○ Yes

Persistent or recurrent experiences of either or both depersonalization or derealization:

 • **Depersonalization** is characterized by experiencing the self as strange or unreal, or feeling detached from, or as though one were an outside observer of, one's thoughts, feelings, sensations, body, or actions. Depersonalization may take the form of emotional and/or physical numbing, a sense of watching oneself from a distance or "being in a play", or perceptual alterations (e.g., a distorted sense of time).

 • **Derealization** is characterized by experiencing other persons, objects, or the world as strange or unreal (e.g., dreamlike, distant, foggy, lifeless, colourless, or visually distorted) or feeling detached from one's surroundings.

DP-DR Disorder, 2nd Essential Feature　　　　○ Unclear　　○ No　　○ Yes

During experiences of depersonalization or derealization, reality testing remains intact. The experiences are not associated with delusions or beliefs that the individual is being controlled by external persons or forces.

DP-DR Disorder, 3rd Essential Feature　　　　○ Unclear　　○ No　　○ Yes

The symptoms are not better accounted for by another mental disorder (e.g., Post-Traumatic Stress Disorder, an Anxiety or Fear-Related Disorder, another Dissociative Disorder, Personality Disorder).

DP-DR Disorder, 4th Essential Feature　　　　○ Unclear　　○ No　　○ Yes

The symptoms are not due to the effect of a substance or medication on the central nervous system, including withdrawal effects, and are not due to a Disease of the Nervous System (e.g., temporal lobe epilepsy) or to head trauma.

DP-DR Disorder, 5th Essential Feature　　　　○ Unclear　　○ No　　○ Yes

The symptoms result in significant distress or significant impairment in personal, family, social, educational, occupational or other important areas of functioning. If functioning is maintained, it is only through significant additional effort.

ICD-11 DISSOCIATIVE IDENTITY DISORDER: ESSENTIAL FEATURES

DID, 1ˢᵗ Essential Feature   ○ Unclear   ○ No   ○ Yes

Disruption of identity characterized by the presence of two or more distinct personality states (dissociative identities), involving marked discontinuities in the sense of self and agency. Each personality state includes its own pattern of experiencing, perceiving, conceiving, and relating to self, the body, and the environment.

DID, 2ⁿᵈ Essential Feature   ○ Unclear   ○ No   ○ Yes

At least two distinct personality states recurrently take executive control of the individual's consciousness and functioning in interacting with others or with the environment, such as in the performance of specific aspects of daily life (e.g., parenting, work), or in response to specific situations (e.g., those that are perceived as threatening).

DID, 3ʳᵈ Essential Feature   ○ Unclear   ○ No   ○ Yes

Changes in personality state are accompanied by related alterations in sensation, perception, affect, cognition, memory, motor control, and behavior. There are typically episodes of amnesia inconsistent with ordinary forgetting, which may be severe.

DID, 4ᵗʰ Essential Feature   ○ Unclear   ○ No   ○ Yes

The symptoms are not better accounted for by another mental disorder (e.g., Schizophrenia or another primary psychotic disorder).

DID, 5ᵗʰ Essential Feature   ○ Unclear   ○ No   ○ Yes

The symptoms are not due to the effect of a substance or medication on the central nervous system, including withdrawal effects (e.g., blackouts or chaotic behavior during substance intoxication), and are not due to a Disease of the Nervous System (e.g., complex partial seizures) or to a Sleep-Wake disorder (e.g., symptoms occur during hypnagogic or hypnopompic states).

DID, 6ᵗʰ Essential Feature   ○ Unclear   ○ No   ○ Yes

The symptoms result in significant impairment in personal, family, social, educational, occupational or other important areas of functioning. If functioning is maintained, it is only through significant additional effort.

ICD-11 PARTIAL DID:
ESSENTIAL FEATURES

Partial DID, 1st Essential Feature   ○ Unclear   ○ No   ○ Yes

Disruption of identity characterized by the experience of two or more distinct personality states (dissociative identities), involving discontinuities in the sense of self and agency. Each personality state includes its own pattern of experiencing, perceiving, conceiving, and relating to self, the body, and the environment.

Partial DID, 2nd Essential Feature   ○ Unclear   ○ No   ○ Yes

One personality state is dominant and functions in daily life (e.g., parenting, work), but is intruded upon by one or more non-dominant personality states (dissociative intrusions). These intrusions may be cognitive (intruding thoughts), affective (intruding affects such as fear, anger, or shame), perceptual (e.g., intruding voices, fleeting visual perceptions, sensations such as being touched), motor (e.g., involuntary movements of an arm), or behavioral (e.g., an action that lacks a sense of agency or ownership). These experiences are experienced as interfering with the functioning of the dominant personality state and are typically aversive.

Partial DID, 3rd Essential Feature   ○ Unclear   ○ No   ○ Yes

The non-dominant personality states do not recurrently take executive control of the individual's consciousness and functioning to the extent that they perform in specific aspects of daily life (e.g., parenting, work). However, there may be occasional, limited and transient episodes in which a distinct personality state assumes executive control to engage in circumscribed behaviors (e.g., in response to extreme emotional states or during episodes of self-harm or the reenactment of traumatic memories).

Partial DID, 4th Essential Feature   ○ Unclear   ○ No   ○ Yes

The symptoms are not better accounted for by another mental disorder (e.g., Schizophrenia or another primary psychotic disorder).

Partial DID, 5th Essential Feature   ○ Unclear   ○ No   ○ Yes

The symptoms are not due to the effect of a substance or medication on the central nervous system, including withdrawal effects (e.g., blackouts or chaotic behavior during substance intoxication), and are not due to a Disease of the Nervous System (e.g., complex partial seizures) or to a Sleep-Wake disorder (e.g., symptoms occur during hypnagogic or hypnopompic states).

Partial DID, 6th Essential Feature   ○ Unclear   ○ No   ○ Yes

The symptoms result in significant impairment in personal, family, social, educational, occupational or other important areas of functioning. If functioning is maintained, it is only through significant additional effort.

ICD-11 OTHER SPECIFIED DISSOCIATIVE DISORDER (OSDD): ESSENTIAL FEATURES

OSDD, 1ˢᵗ Essential Feature   ○ Unclear   ○ No   ○ Yes

The presentation is characterized by symptoms that share primary clinical features with other Dissociative Disorders (i.e., involuntary disruption or discontinuity in the normal integration of one or more of the following: identity, sensations, perceptions, affects, thoughts, memories, control over bodily movements, or behavior).

OSDD, 2ⁿᵈ Essential Feature   ○ Unclear   ○ No   ○ Yes

The symptoms do not fulfil the diagnostic requirements of any of the other disorders in the grouping of Dissociative Disorders.

OSDD, 3ʳᵈ Essential Feature   ○ Unclear   ○ No   ○ Yes

The symptoms are not better accounted for by another mental disorder (e.g., Post-Traumatic Stress Disorder, Complex Post-Traumatic Stress Disorder, Schizophrenia, Bipolar Disorders).

OSDD, 4ᵗʰ Essential Feature   ○ Unclear   ○ No   ○ Yes

The symptoms are involuntary and unwanted and are not accepted as a part of a collective cultural or religious practice.

OSDD, 5ᵗʰ Essential Feature   ○ Unclear   ○ No   ○ Yes

The symptoms are not due to the effect of a substance or medication on the central nervous system, including withdrawal effects (e.g., blackouts or chaotic behavior during substance intoxication), and are not due to a Disease of the Nervous System (e.g., complex partial seizures), a Sleep-Wake disorder (e.g., symptoms occur during hypnagogic or hypnopompic states), head trauma, or another medical condition.

OSDD, 6ᵗʰ Essential Feature   ○ Unclear   ○ No   ○ Yes

The symptoms result in significant distress or significant impairment in personal, family, social, educational, occupational or other important areas of functioning. If functioning is maintained, it is only through significant additional effort.

ICD-11 TRANCE DISORDER:
ESSENTIAL FEATURES

OSDD, 1st Essential Feature   ⭕ Unclear   ⭕ No   ⭕ Yes

Occurrence of a trance state in which there is a marked alteration in the individual's state of consciousness or a loss of the individual's normal sense of personal identity, characterized by both of the following:

- Narrowing of awareness of immediate surroundings or unusually narrow and selective focusing on specific environmental stimuli; and

- Restriction of movements, postures, and speech to repetition of a small repertoire that is experienced as being outside of one's control.

OSDD, 2nd Essential Feature   ⭕ Unclear   ⭕ No   ⭕ Yes

The trance state is not characterized by the experience of being replaced by an alternate identity.

OSDD, 3rd Essential Feature   ⭕ Unclear   ⭕ No   ⭕ Yes

Trance episodes are recurrent or, if the diagnosis is based on a single episode, the episode has lasted for at least several days.

OSDD, 4th Essential Feature   ⭕ Unclear   ⭕ No   ⭕ Yes

The trance state is involuntary and unwanted and is not accepted as a part of a collective cultural or religious practice.

OSDD, 5th Essential Feature   ⭕ Unclear   ⭕ No   ⭕ Yes

The symptoms are not due to the effects of a substance or medication on the central nervous system (including withdrawal effects), exhaustion, or to hypnagogic or hypnopompic states, and are not due to a Disease of the Nervous System (e.g., complex partial seizures), head trauma, or a Sleep-Wake Disorder.

OSDD, 6th Essential Feature   ⭕ Unclear   ⭕ No   ⭕ Yes

The symptoms result in significant distress or significant impairment in personal, family, social, educational, occupational or other important areas of functioning. If functioning is maintained, it is only through significant additional effort.

ICD-11 POSSESSION TRANCE DISORDER: ESSENTIAL FEATURES

OSDD, 1ˢᵗ Essential Feature   ○ Unclear   ○ No   ○ Yes
Occurrence of a trance state in which there is a marked alteration in the individual's state of consciousness and the individual's normal sense of personal identity is replaced by an external "possessing" identity. The trance state is characterized by behaviors or movements that are experienced as being controlled by the possessing agent.

OSDD, 2ⁿᵈ Essential Feature   ○ Unclear   ○ No   ○ Yes
Trance episodes are attributed to the influence of an external "possessing" spirit, power, deity or other spiritual entity.

OSDD, 3ʳᵈ Essential Feature   ○ Unclear   ○ No   ○ Yes
Trance episodes are recurrent or, if the diagnosis is based on a single episode, the episode has lasted for at least several days.

OSDD, 4ᵗʰ Essential Feature   ○ Unclear   ○ No   ○ Yes
The possession trance state is involuntary and unwanted and is not accepted as a part of a collective cultural or religious practice.

OSDD, 5ᵗʰ Essential Feature   ○ Unclear   ○ No   ○ Yes
The symptoms are not due to the effect of a substance or medication on the central nervous system (including withdrawal effects), exhaustion, or to hypnagogic or hypnopompic states, and are not due to a Disease of the Nervous System (e.g., complex partial seizures) or a Sleep-Wake Disorder.

OSDD, 6ᵗʰ Essential Feature   ○ Unclear   ○ No   ○ Yes
The symptoms result in significant distress or impairment in personal, family, social, educational, occupational or other important areas of functioning. If functioning is maintained, it is only through significant additional effort.

ICD-11 DISSOCIATIVE NEUROLOGICAL SYMPTOM DISORDER: ESSENTIAL FEATURES

Dissociative Neurological Symptom Disorder (SD),
1st Essential Feature   O Unclear   O No   O Yes
Involuntary disruption or discontinuity in the normal integration of motor, sensory, or cognitive functions, lasting at least several hours.

Dissociative Neurological SD, 2nd Essential Feature   O Unclear   O No   O Yes
Clinical findings are not consistent with a recognized Disease of the Nervous System (e.g., a stroke) or another medical condition (e.g., a head injury).

Dissociative Neurological SD, 3rd Essential Feature   O Unclear   O No   O Yes
The symptoms do not occur exclusively during episodes of Trance Disorder, Possession Trance Disorder, Dissociative Identity Disorder, or Partial Dissociative Identity Disorder.

Dissociative Neurological SD, 4th Essential Feature   O Unclear   O No   O Yes
The symptoms are not due to the effect of a substance or medication on the central nervous system, including withdrawal effects, do not occur exclusively during hypnagogic or hypnopompic states, and are not due to a Sleep-Wake disorder (e.g., Sleep-Related Rhythmic Movement Disorder, Recurrent isolated sleep paralysis).

Dissociative Neurological SD, 5th Essential Feature   O Unclear   O No   O Yes
The symptoms are not better accounted for by another mental disorder (e.g., Schizophrenia or another primary psychotic disorder, Post-Traumatic Stress Disorder).

Dissociative Neurological SD, 6th Essential Feature   O Unclear   O No   O Yes
The symptoms result in significant impairment in personal, family, social, educational, occupational or other important areas of functioning.

ICD-11 DISSOCIATIVE NEUROLOGICAL SYMPTOM DISORDER: SYMPTOM QUALIFIERS

Specific presenting symptoms in Dissociative Neurological Symptom Disorder may be identified using the following symptom qualifiers. Multiple qualifiers may be assigned as necessary to describe the clinical presentation.

—with visual disturbance: ○ Unclear   ○ No   ○ Yes
Characterized by visual symptoms such as blindness, tunnel vision, diplopia, visual distortions or hallucinations.

—with auditory disturbance: ○ Unclear   ○ No   ○ Yes
Characterized by auditory symptoms such as loss of hearing or auditory hallucinations.

—with vertigo or dizziness: ○ Unclear   ○ No   ○ Yes
Characterized by a sensation of spinning while stationary (vertigo) or dizziness.

—with other sensory disturbance: ○ Unclear   ○ No   ○ Yes
Characterized by sensory symptoms not identified in other specific categories in this grouping such as numbness, tightness, tingling, burning, pain, or other symptoms related to touch, smell, taste, balance, proprioception, kinesthesia, or thermoception.

—with non-epileptic seizures: ○ Unclear   ○ No   ○ Yes
Characterized by a symptomatic presentation of seizures or convulsions.

—with speech disturbance: ○ Unclear   ○ No   ○ Yes
Characterized by symptoms such as difficulty with speaking (dysphonia), loss of the ability to speak (aphonia) or difficult or unclear articulation of speech (dysarthria).

—with paresis or weakness: ○ Unclear   ○ No   ○ Yes
Characterized by a difficulty or inability to intentionally move parts of the body or to coordinate movements.

—with gait disturbance: ○ Unclear   ○ No   ○ Yes
Characterized by symptoms involving the individual's ability or manner of walking, including ataxia and the inability to stand unaided.

—with movement disturbance: ○ Unclear   ○ No   ○ Yes
Characterized by symptoms such as chorea, myoclonus, tremor, dystonia, facial spasm, parkinsonism, or dyskinesia.

—with cognitive symptoms: ○ Unclear   ○ No   ○ Yes
Characterized by impaired cognitive performance in memory, language or other cognitive domains that is internally inconsistent.

—with other specified motor, sensory, or cognitive symptoms   ○ Unclear   ○ No   ○ Yes

APPENDIX 3B:
DSM-5-TR DIAGNOSTIC CRITERIA
FOR THE DISSOCIATIVE DISORDERS

DSM-5-TR DIAGNOSTIC CRITERIA FOR THE DISSOCIATIVE DISORDERS

The information gleaned in the SCID-D interview can be used to determine which DSM dissociative disorder criteria have been fulfilled, and consequently which particular dissociative disorder diagnosis, if any, is present. Table 1 below lists the various dissociative disorders as classified in DSM-5, along with the page numbers which list the corresponding DSM criteria.

Before considering the DSM diagnostic criteria, it is often helpful to first complete Section A of the *SCID-D Summary Scoresheet* (see Appendix 4B, page 163), which rates the severity of each of the five SCID-D symptoms. Completing that section of the *Scoresheet* beforehand will inform the likely DSM diagnosis (e.g., by identifying whether moderate-to-severe levels of amnesia co-occur with high levels of several other SCID-D symptoms, suggesting a DID or OSDD diagnosis, or alternatively if amnesia is the only elevated symptom, suggesting a Dissociative Amnesia diagnosis). It is also helpful, before considering the DSM diagnostic criteria, to compare your client's SCID-D symptom severity scores to profile norms of research participants with confirmed dissociative disorders (see Appendix 4C, page 167 for a graphical representation of averaged profiles of SCID-D symptom severity scores for previous research participants with confirmed DID or OSDD [née DDNOS] diagnosis). For further discussion of the dissociative symptom profiles for each of the dissociative disorders, see the *Interviewer's Guide to the SCID-D.*

After completing the dissociative symptoms severity on the *SCID-D Summary Scoresheet* as recommended above, select the DSM dissociative disorder in Table 1 which you believe the client has, refer to the corresponding page mentioned in the table, and rate the presence or absence of the specific diagnostic features to determine if the client's presentation meets the criteria listed.

Table 1: Diagnosing Dissociative Disorders Based on DSM-5-TR

Dissociative Disorder	DSM-5-TR Diagnostic Criteria
Dissociative Amnesia	page 154
Depersonalization/Derealization Disorder	page 155
Dissociative Identity Disorder	page 156
Other Specified Dissociative Disorder	page 157
Unspecified Dissociative Disorder	page 158

DSM-5-TR CRITERIA:
DISSOCIATIVE AMNESIA

Dissociative Amnesia Criterion A   ○ Unclear   ○ No   ○ Yes

An inability to recall important autobiographical information, usually of a traumatic or stressful nature, that is inconsistent with ordinary forgetting. Note: Dissociative Amnesia most often consists of localized or selective amnesia for a specific event(s); or generalized amnesia for identity and life history.

Dissociative Amnesia Criterion B   ○ Unclear   ○ No   ○ Yes

The symptoms cause clinically significant distress or impairment in social, occupational, or other important areas of functioning.

Dissociative Amnesia Criterion C   ○ Unclear   ○ No   ○ Yes

The disturbance is not attributable to the physiological effects of a substance (e.g., alcohol or other drug of abuse, a medication) or a neurological or other medical condition (e.g., partial complex seizures, transient global amnesia, sequelae of a closed head injury/traumatic brain injury, other neurological condition).

Dissociative Amnesia Criterion D   ○ Unclear   ○ No   ○ Yes

The disturbance is not better explained by dissociative identity disorder, posttraumatic stress disorder, acute stress disorder, somatic symptom disorder, or major or mild neurocognitive disorder.

Specify if: With dissociative fugue   ○ Unclear   ○ No   ○ Yes

Apparently purposeful travel or bewildered wandering that is associated with amnesia for identity or for other important autobiographical information.

DSM-5-TR CRITERIA: DEPERSONALIZATION/DEREALIZATION DISORDER

Depersonalization/Derealization Disorder Criterion A   ○ Unclear   ○ No   ○ Yes
The presence of persistent or recurrent experiences of depersonalization, derealization, or both:

1. **Depersonalization**: Experiences of unreality, detachment, or being an outside observer with respect to one's thoughts, feelings, sensations, body, or actions (e.g., perceptual alterations, distorted sense of time, unreal or absent self, emotional and/or physical numbing).

2. **Derealization**: Experiences of unreality or detachment with respect to surroundings (e.g., individuals or objects are experienced as unreal, dreamlike, foggy, lifeless, or visually distorted).

Depersonalization/Derealization Disorder Criterion B   ○ Unclear   ○ No   ○ Yes
During the depersonalization or derealization experiences, reality testing remains intact.

Depersonalization/Derealization Disorder Criterion C   ○ Unclear   ○ No   ○ Yes
The symptoms cause clinically significant distress or impairment in social, occupational, or other important areas of functioning.

Depersonalization/Derealization Disorder Criterion D   ○ Unclear   ○ No   ○ Yes
The disturbance is not attributable to the physiological effects of a substance (e.g., a drug of abuse, a medication) or another medical condition (e.g., seizures).

Depersonalization/Derealization Disorder Criterion E   ○ Unclear   ○ No   ○ Yes
The disturbance is not better explained by another mental disorder, such as schizophrenia, panic disorder, major depressive disorder, acute stress disorder, posttraumatic stress disorder, or another dissociative disorder.

DSM-5-TR CRITERIA:
DISSOCIATIVE IDENTITY DISORDER

Dissociative Identity Disorder Criterion A   ○ Unclear   ○ No   ○ Yes

Disruption of identity characterized by two or more distinct personality states, which may be described in some cultures as an experience of possession. The disruption in identity involves marked discontinuity in sense of self and sense of agency, accompanied by related alterations in affect, behavior, consciousness, memory, perception, cognition, and/or sensory-motor functioning. These signs and symptoms may be observed by others or reported by the individual.

Dissociative Identity Disorder Criterion B   ○ Unclear   ○ No   ○ Yes

Recurrent gaps in the recall of everyday events, important personal information, and/or traumatic events that are inconsistent with ordinary forgetting.

Dissociative Identity Disorder Criterion C   ○ Unclear   ○ No   ○ Yes

The symptoms cause clinically significant distress or impairment in social, occupational, or other important areas of functioning.

Dissociative Identity Disorder Criterion D   ○ Unclear   ○ No   ○ Yes

The disturbance is not a normal part of a broadly accepted cultural or religious practice.

Dissociative Identity Disorder Criterion E   ○ Unclear   ○ No   ○ Yes

The symptoms are not attributable to the physiological effects of a substance (e.g., blackouts or chaotic behavior during alcohol intoxication) or another medical condition (e.g., complex partial seizures).

DSM-5-TR CRITERIA:
OTHER SPECIFIED DISSOCIATIVE DISORDER

Other Specified Dissociative Disorder   ○ Unclear   ○ No   ○ Yes

This category applies to presentations in which symptoms characteristic of a dissociative disorder that cause clinically significant distress or impairment in social, occupational, or other important areas of functioning predominate but do not meet full criteria for any of the disorders in the dissociative disorders diagnostic class. The other specified dissociative disorder category is used in situations in which the clinician chooses to communicate the specific reason that the presentation does not meet the criteria for any specific dissociative disorder. Examples of presentation that can be specified using the "otherwise specified" designation include:

1. Chronic and recurrent syndromes of mixed dissociative symptoms   ○ Unclear   ○ No   ○ Yes

This category includes identity disturbance associated with less-than-marked discontinuities in sense of self and agency, or alterations in identity or episodes of possession in an individual who reports no dissociative amnesia.

2. Identity disturbance due to prolonged and intense coercive persuasion   ○ Unclear   ○ No   ○ Yes

Individuals subjected to intense coercive persuasion (e.g., brainwashing, thought reform, indoctrination while captive, torture, long-term political imprisonment, recruitment by sects/cults or by terror organizations) may present with prolonged changes in, or conscious questioning of, their identity.

3. Acute dissociative reactions to stressful events   ○ Unclear   ○ No   ○ Yes

This category is for acute, transient conditions that typically last less than 1 month, and sometimes only a few hours or days. These conditions are characterized by constriction of consciousness; depersonalization; derealization; perceptual disturbances (e.g., time slowing, macropsia); micro-amnesias; transient stupor; and/or alterations in sensory-motor functioning (e.g., analgesia, paralysis).

4. Dissociative trance   ○ Unclear   ○ No   ○ Yes

The condition is characterized by an acute narrowing or complete loss of awareness of immediate surroundings that manifests as profound unresponsiveness or insensitivity to environmental stimuli. The unresponsiveness may be accompanied by minor stereotyped behaviors (e.g., finger movements) of which the individual is unaware and/or that he/she cannot control, as well as transient paralysis or loss of consciousness. The dissociative trance is not a normal part of a broadly accepted collective cultural or religious practice.

DSM-5-TR CRITERIA:
UNSPECIFIED DISSOCIATIVE DISORDER

Unspecified Dissociative Disorder   ○ Unclear   ○ No   ○ Yes

This category applies to presentations in which symptoms characteristic of a dissociative disorder that cause clinically significant distress or impairment in social, occupational, or other important areas of functioning predominate but do not meet the full criteria for any of the disorders in the dissociative disorders diagnostic class. This category is used in situations in which the clinician chooses *not* to specify the reason that the criteria are not met for a specific dissociative disorder, and includes presentations for which there is insufficient information to make a more specific diagnosis (e.g., in emergency room setting).

APPENDIX 4A:
SUMMARY SCORESHEET
(WITH ICD-11 DIAGNOSES)

Client's Identifier _____   Date _____

Interviewer _____   Total SCID-D Score _____

SCID-D SUMMARY SCORESHEET* (ICD-11)

A. Components of Dissociation	Severity	Occurs With Alcohol/Drugs?
Amnesia	1 ❑ Absent 2 ❑ Mild 3 ❑ Moderate 4 ❑ Severe	❑ Unclear ❑ Only with substance use ❑ Sometimes ❑ Not associated
Depersonalization	1 ❑ Absent 2 ❑ Mild 3 ❑ Moderate 4 ❑ Severe	❑ Unclear ❑ Only with substance use ❑ Sometimes ❑ Not associated
Derealization	1 ❑ Absent 2 ❑ Mild 3 ❑ Moderate 4 ❑ Severe	❑ Unclear ❑ Only with substance use ❑ Sometimes ❑ Not associated
Identity Confusion	1 ❑ Absent 2 ❑ Mild 3 ❑ Moderate 4 ❑ Severe	❑ Unclear ❑ Only with substance use ❑ Sometimes ❑ Not associated
Identity Alteration	1 ❑ Absent 2 ❑ Mild 3 ❑ Moderate 4 ❑ Severe	❑ Unclear ❑ Only with substance use ❑ Sometimes ❑ Not associated
B. Total SCID-D Score	_____	
C. Diagnostic Conclusion	❑ No Dissociative Disorder ❑ Meets criteria for a Dissociative Disorder ❑ Presently ❑ Past episode	
D. Type of Dissociative Disorder (ICD-11)	❑ Dissociative Amnesia ❑ Depersonalization-Derealization Disorder ❑ Dissociative Identity Disorder ❑ Partial Dissociative Identity Disorder ❑ Trance Disorder ❑ Possession Trance Disorder ❑ Dissociative Neurological Symptom Disorder ❑ Other Specified Dissociative Disorder ❑ Unspecified Dissociative Disorder ❑ Secondary Dissociative Syndrome	

Cite as: Steinberg M: *The SCID-D Interview: Dissociation Assessment in Therapy, Forensics, and Research.* Washington, DC, American Psychiatric Association Publishing, 2023

SCID-D SUMMARY SCORESHEET* (ICD-11)

E. If client has Dissociative Neurological Symptom Disorder, note symptom qualifier:	With: ❑ visual disturbance ❑ paresis or weakness ❑ auditory disturbance ❑ gait disturbance ❑ vertigo or dizziness ❑ movement disturbance ❑ other sensory disturbance ❑ cognitive symptoms ❑ non-epileptic seizures ❑ other specified motor, sensory, or ❑ speech disturbance cognitive symptoms
F. Exclusion Factors Summary *(check all that apply)*	❑ No reason to exclude dissociative disorder diagnosis ❑ Symptom severity does not rise to level of a dissociative disorder ❑ Symptoms are better explained by another psychiatric disorder (Optional: Specify other psychiatric disorder suspected: _____) ❑ Dissociative symptoms occur <u>only</u> with drugs or alcohol use ❑ Dissociative symptoms are due to other organic or medical condition ❑ Suspect feigning or malingering
G. Personality States Summary	❑ Inadequate information ❑ Lacks evidence of 2 or more personality states ❑ Suspect 2 or more personality states, but distinctness is unclear ❑ Has 2 or more distinct personality states (accompanied by related alterations in affect, memory, behavior, cognition, and/or sensory-motor functioning)
H. Shifts in Executive Control/Agency Summary	❑ Inadequate information ❑ Lacks evidence of shifts in executive control ❑ Shifts in control seem less-than-marked ❑ Marked shifts in executive control

*Severity ratings of the five SCID-D components of dissociation should be performed using the guidelines and the Severity Rating Definitions described in the *Interviewer's Guide to the SCID-D* (Washington, DC, American Psychiatric Association Publishing, 1993, under development).

APPENDIX 4B:
SUMMARY SCORESHEET
(WITH DSM-5-TR DIAGNOSES)

Client's Identifier _____   Date _____

Interviewer _____   Total SCID-D Score _____

SCID-D SUMMARY SCORESHEET* (DSM-5-TR)

A. Components of Dissociation	Severity	Occurs With Alcohol/Drugs?
Amnesia	1 ❑ Absent 2 ❑ Mild 3 ❑ Moderate 4 ❑ Severe	❑ Unclear ❑ Only with substance use ❑ Sometimes ❑ Not associated
Depersonalization	1 ❑ Absent 2 ❑ Mild 3 ❑ Moderate 4 ❑ Severe	❑ Unclear ❑ Only with substance use ❑ Sometimes ❑ Not associated
Derealization	1 ❑ Absent 2 ❑ Mild 3 ❑ Moderate 4 ❑ Severe	❑ Unclear ❑ Only with substance use ❑ Sometimes ❑ Not associated
Identity Confusion	1 ❑ Absent 2 ❑ Mild 3 ❑ Moderate 4 ❑ Severe	❑ Unclear ❑ Only with substance use ❑ Sometimes ❑ Not associated
Identity Alteration	1 ❑ Absent 2 ❑ Mild 3 ❑ Moderate 4 ❑ Severe	❑ Unclear ❑ Only with substance use ❑ Sometimes ❑ Not associated
B. Total SCID-D Score	_____	
C. Diagnostic Conclusion	❑ No dissociative disorder ❑ Meets criteria for a dissociative disorder ❑ Presently ❑ Past episode	
D. Type of Dissociative Disorder (DSM-5-TR)	❑ Dissociative Amnesia ❑ With dissociative fugue ❑ Depersonalization-Derealization Disorder ❑ Dissociative Identity Disorder ❑ Other Specified Dissociative Disorder (OSDD) ❑ Unspecified Dissociative Disorder	

Cite as: Steinberg M: The SCID-D Interview: Dissociation Assessment in Therapy, Forensics, and Research. Washington, DC, American Psychiatric Association Publishing, 2023

SCID-D SUMMARY SCORESHEET* (DSM-5-TR)

E. If the client meets criteria for OSDD, note reason	❑ Chronic and recurrent syndromes of mixed dissociative symptoms ❑ Identity disturbance due to prolonged and intense coercive persuasion ❑ Acute dissociative reactions to stressful events ❑ Dissociative trance
F. Exclusion Factors Summary *(check all that apply)*	❑ No reason to exclude dissociative disorder diagnosis ❑ Symptom severity does not rise to level of a dissociative disorder ❑ Symptoms are better explained by another psychiatric disorder (Optional: Specify other psychiatric disorder suspected: _____) ❑ Dissociative symptoms occur only with drugs or alcohol use ❑ Dissociative symptoms are due to other organic or medical condition ❑ Suspect feigning or malingering
G. Personality States Summary	❑ Inadequate information ❑ Lacks evidence of 2 or more personality states ❑ Suspect 2 or more personality states, but distinctness is unclear ❑ Has 2 or more distinct personality states (accompanied by related alterations in affect, memory, behavior, cognition, and/or sensory-motor functioning)
H. Shifts in Executive Control/Agency Summary	❑ Inadequate information ❑ Lacks evidence of shifts in executive control ❑ Shifts in control seem less-than-marked ❑ Marked shifts in executive control

*Severity ratings of the five SCID-D components of dissociation should be performed using the guidelines and the Severity Rating Definitions described in the *Interviewer's Guide to the SCID-D* (Washington, DC, American Psychiatric Association Publishing, 1993, under development).

APPENDIX 4C:
CHARTING THE CLIENT'S SCID-D PROFILE

Client's Identifier _____ Date _____

Interviewer _____ Total SCID-D Score _____

CHARTING THE CLIENT'S SCID-D PROFILE

To create a graphical representation of SCID-D Severity Scores, also known as a *symptom profile*, plot your client's severity scores for each of the five SCID-D components of dissociation and then draw a line connecting each score. Compare this to the standard graph below, which charts profiles of complex dissociative disorders, other psychiatric disorders, and normal controls based on mean SCID-D dissociative symptom severity scores from research studies in Germany, the Netherlands, Switzerland, Turkey, the United Kingdom, and the United States. See Appendix 2 for other standard profiles.

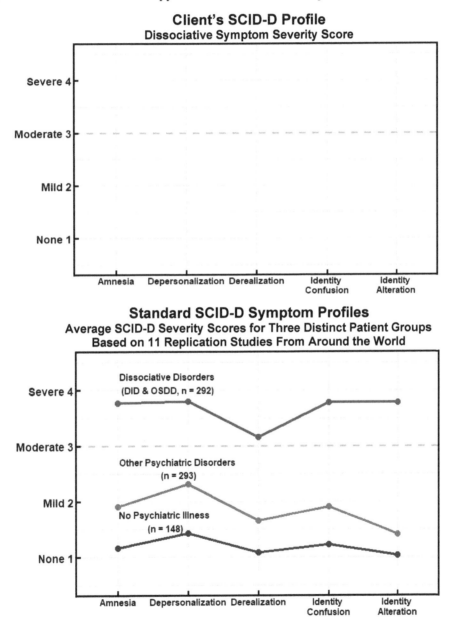

DID = Dissociative Identity Disorder; DDNOS = Dissociative Disorder Not Otherwise Specified (DSM-IV-R). *Note:* DDNOS (DSM-IV-R) is similar to OSDD (Other Specified Dissociative Disorder), Example 1 (DSM-5). Partial DID (ICD-11) may have a similar dissociation profile to OSDD, Example 1 and DID.

See *Interviewer's Guide to the SCID-D* for citations to studies included in the above symptom profiles.

Cite as: Steinberg M: The SCID-D Interview: Dissociation Assessment in Therapy, Forensics, and Research. Washington, DC, American Psychiatric Association Publishing, 2023